AF683646

The Cycle of Offense
A Framework for Treating Adolescent Sexual Offenders

Ineke F. Way, A.C.S.W. and Stephen D. Spieker, L.P.C.

Jalice Publishers
Notre Dame, Indiana

The Cycle of Offense: A Framework for Treating Adolescent Sexual Offenders.

Published by Jalice Publishers
P.O. Box 455
Notre Dame, IN 46556

219/232-9534

Library of Congress Cataloging-in-Publication Data

The cycle of offense: A framework for treating adolescent sexual offenders by Ineke F. Way & Stephen D. Spieker.

ISBN 0-9627375-7-7

1. Teenage sex offenders. I. Way, Ineke F. II. Spieker, Stephen D.

Printed in the United States of America.
International Standard Book Number: 0-9627375-7-7
Library of Congress Card Number: 96-78274

DEDICATION

This book is dedicated to children and adults who were sexually abused and who demonstrate courage and dignity in their growing and thriving. It is our intention to honor their lives through this contribution to preventing further abuse.

We also dedicate this book to Fay Honey Knopp, whose faithful work in sexual offender treatment program development and research has furthered our ability to intervene effectively with sexual offenders.

ACKNOWLEDGEMENTS

It is with great appreciation that we acknowledge the assistance and support of colleagues and family members who offered input, encouragement, and energy during the writing of this book:

To Gail D. Ryan for her work in advancing knowledge through the Adolescent Perpetrator Network, and for her review and valuable input on the manuscript;

To our editor, Thomas Balthazor, who guided the writing of this manuscript and gave input and valuable feedback on the many drafts.

To colleagues who read many versions of the manuscript in its various stages: Stella Chowdhury, Jeanine Curtis, Christopher Dryer, Ron Grooters, David Loeker, Tobi Sisman, Ron Smith, and Ginny VanderZee;

To Ronald L. Grooters, who collaborated in writing Chapters 5 and 6;

To Michael Kruk, for assistance with the literature search;

To Steve's wife, Liz, and children, Katy, Kyle, Keith, and Kurt, for their patience and encouragement. Thank you!

To Liz Visser, for her expertise in editing the manuscript;

To Ellen Balthazor for proof reading the final manuscript.

To David Spieker and John and Cheryl Washburn for valuable computer assistance;

It is our hope that this book can be yet another tool in the important task of effective intervention in the cycle of sexual abuse.

Table of Contents

Chapter 1
Significance of Adolescent Sexual Offense

In the last fifteen years, numerous authors have documented the significance of adolescent sexual perpetration and the need for an effective therapeutic response to halt the progression into adult sexual offenses (Becker, Cunningham-Rathner, & Kaplan, 1986; Davis & Leitenberg, 1987; National Task Force on Juvenile Sexual Offending, 1993; Ryan & Lane, 1991). The National Task Force on Juvenile Sexual Offending (1993) emphasizes the importance of a comprehensive community response to adolescent sexual offense that includes specialized treatment within a continuum of care. A broad understanding of the context of sexual offense serves as a foundation for planning and implementing effective treatment intervention with adolescents who have sexually offended. This chapter discusses the significance of adolescent sexual offense and presents incidence statistics, outlines the adolescent sexual offense histories of adult sexual offenders, and discusses the potential progression from victim to victimizer.

Incidence

An adolescent sexual offender is commonly defined as "a minor who commits any sexual act with a person of any age 1) against the victim's will, 2) without consent, or 3) in an aggressive, exploitive, or threatening manner" (Ryan & Lane, 1991, p. 3). The report of the National Task Force on Juvenile Sexual Offending (1993) adds, "It is the nature of the relationship; the equality or inequality of the participants; presence of exploitation, coercion, and control; manipulation; and the abuse of power combined with sexual behavior which constitutes sexual abuse" (p. 6).

Research studies primarily describe the characteristics of adolescents who have sexually offended, and conclusive statistics on the incidence of adolescent sexual offending are limited (Ryan & Lane, 1991). Research indicates that approximately 20 percent of all rapes and 30 to 50 percent of all child molestations are committed by adolescents (Barbaree, Hudson, & Seto, 1993), and 56 to 57 percent of boys who are molested are assaulted by an adolescent (Rogers & Tremaine, 1984; Showers, Farber, Joseph, Oshins, & Johnson, 1983). The federal Uniform Crime Reports documented a doubling in arrests of adolescents for forcible rape, from 10.9 per 100,000 in 1965 to 21.9 per 100,000 in 1990 (1991). For 1993, the Uniform Crime Reports showed that 16 percent of forcible rapes and 19 percent of all other sexual offenses (excluding forcible rape and prostitution) were committed by juveniles (1993). Becker & Kaplan (1988) found that approximately 20 percent of rapes and roughly 40 percent of child sexual abuse cases were perpetrated by adolescents. It must be recognized that adolescent sexual offenses are underreported (Knopp, 1984), and that statistics reflect only those crimes brought to the attention of the criminal justice system.

Youth of color are over-represented in criminal justice statistics, but research indicates that these youth do not have a greater involvement in serious criminal behavior overall (Krisberg, Schwartz, Fishman, Eisikovits, Guttman, & Joe, 1987; McGarrell, 1993; Schwartz, 1989). They are, however, significantly more likely than white youths to be arrested and then charged with more serious offenses (Bridges, Conley, Beretta, Engen, Price-Spratlen, Rankin, & Steen, 1993; Krisberg, et al., 1987). In 1990, 53 percent of the juveniles arrested for rape were white, 46 percent were black, and 2 percent were of other races (Uniform Crime Reports, 1991). Marshall, Laws, & Barbaree (1990) studied 561 adolescent and adult sexual offenders, ages 13 to 76, and found that the ethnic distribution of these offenders was consistent with the population makeup in the cities where the research was conducted. Research also suggests that the overall statistics for juvenile offending may be more a socioeconomic, class-linked issue than a race-linked phenomenon (Huizinga & Elliott, 1987). While caution is critical in interpreting these limited data, and further study is necessary (Finkelhor, Araji, Baron, Browne, Peters, & Wyatt, 1986), sexually abusive behavior clearly occurs in all ethnic groups.

In the last twelve years, there has been increased research on the incidence and dynamics of sexual offenses by female adolescents. Studies indicate that 3 to 20 percent of adolescent sexual offenders are female (Fehrenbach, Smith, Monastersky, & Deisher, 1986; Smith & Israel, 1987; Wasserman & Kappel, 1985). Fehrenbach, et al., (1986) found that fewer than 3 percent of their 305 subjects were female, while Wasserman and Kappel (1985) found 10 percent females in their study of 161 adolescent sexual offenders. In their study of sibling incest offenders, Smith and Israel (1987) found that 20 percent were female. Significant under-representation of sexual offenses by females is suspected, since victims report higher rates of victimization by females than is reflected in the statistics on identified perpetrators (G.D. Ryan, personal communication, June 1996).

Numerous authors have recognized sexually abusive behavior among developmentally disabled youth and have detailed the unique treatment needs of developmentally disabled adolescents. “Most reports state that 10-15% of those who exhibit sexually deviant behavior are handicapped [developmentally disabled]” (Murphy, Coleman, & Haynes, 1983, p. 23). Gilby, Wolf, and Goldberg (1989) report on a study of outpatient and inpatient adolescent sexual offenders at an assessment and treatment center in Ontario. For fourteen months, developmentally disabled adolescents and those of average intelligence were studied, and the two groups showed a similar rate of sexually aggressive behavior. At the same time, developmentally disabled adolescents demonstrated significantly higher levels of such behaviors as public masturbation and exhibitionism (Gilby, et al., 1989).

Griffiths, Quinsey, and Hingsburger (1989) report that developmentally disabled sexual offenders tend to have fewer victims, molest males less often, and demonstrate a greater need for social skill development. Alaska Specialized Education and Training Services (ASETS) in Anchorage has noted the important distinction between deviant arousal and deviant sexual behavior, with the latter being more amenable to change through treatment (Ward, Heffern, Wilcox, McElwee, Dowrick, Brown, Jones, & Johnson, 1992). This research underscores the urgency of formulating effective treatment for developmentally disabled adolescents who have sexually offended.

Adolescent History of Adult Offenders.

Research documents that 43 percent to 80 percent of adult sexual offenders report that they committed their first sexual assault when they were adolescents and that there was frequently no legal system intervention (Abel, Mittelman, & Becker, 1985; Abel, Osborn, & Twigg, 1993; Abel & Rouleau, 1990). Marshall, et al., (1990) report research indicating adult sexual offenders had a lifetime average of 380 sexual offenses. Prentky and Knight (1993) studied adult rapists and child molesters and found that those who had begun sexually offending before age 18 had achieved a lower level of overall competence as adults, including an increased likelihood to engage in antisocial and impulsive behavior. These chilling statistics outline the risk posed by untreated adolescent sexual offenders and affirm the need for therapists to effectively intervene with adolescent sexual offenders. Early intervention and treatment become crucial in order to interrupt the cycle of sexual offending before abusive patterns become ingrained. As Marie Clark (1995) succinctly stated, "If we truly want to stop child abuse, we need to work with adolescent sexual offenders."

Victim to Victimizer Progression

Intervention in adolescent sexual assault is complicated by the reality that many adolescents have experienced sexual or physical abuse, or grown up with violence perpetrated against family members (Ford and Linney, 1995; Kahn and Chambers, 1991; O'Brien, 1989; Smith, 1988). Ford and Linney (1995) studied juvenile child molesters, rapists, violent nonsexual offenders, and status offenders, and found that juvenile child molesters reported significantly more violence within their families and higher rates of physical abuse and sexual victimization in comparison with other offender categories. Studies indicate that between 42 percent and 62 percent of male juvenile sexual offenders report being sexually abused (Kahn & Lafond, 1988; O'Brien, 1989; Worling, 1995).

An even higher incidence of sexual victimization is found when reviewing the histories of female adolescent sexual offenders (Hunter, Lexier, Goodwin,

Browne, & Dennis, 1993; Kahn & Lafond, 1988; Knopp & Lackey, 1987; Mathews, Hunter, & Vuz, 1997). Mathews, Hunter, & Vuz (1997) reported that 77.6% of their sample of 67 female adolescent sexual offenders had themselves been molested, frequently by multiple offenders. Hunter, et al., (1993) reported a study of ten female adolescent sexual offenders and found that eight reported they were physically abused; all stated they were sexually abused. Kahn and Lafond (1988) reported a study of 25 female sexual offenders, all of whom had been sexually abused.

There is a need to not only help prevent adolescent sexual offenders from becoming adult sexual offenders, but also to effectively intervene with children who have been sexually abused so they do not progress into the abuser cycle (Bagley, Wood, & Young, 1994; Ryan, 1989). Lane (1991) notes that adolescents' sexually abusive behavior often begins as early as ages eight or nine. In a study of sexually abusive children under age ten, the SPARK Program in Los Angeles found that 90 percent had themselves been molested (Newsweek, 1992). Ryan (1989) highlights the importance of using lessons learned from sexual offender treatment to effectively treat children who have been sexually abused to resolve their victimization without sexually offending. She details a Dysfunctional Response Cycle experienced by child victims of sexual abuse and urges therapists to create a therapeutic environment that assists child victims in dealing with their issues of powerlessness, helplessness, and vulnerability without relying on retaliatory or compensatory control seeking.

In summary, these concerns demonstrate the importance of intervening effectively with adolescent sexual offenders in order to protect children who are potential victims, assist adolescent sexual offenders to regain maximum healthy functioning, and prevent adolescents from progressing to adult sexual offending. The multiplicity of issues facing adolescent sexual offenders suggests that therapeutic intervention must be focused and intentional if it is to help prevent reoffense.

References

Abel, G.G., Mittelman, M.S., & Becker, J.V. (1985). Sex offenders: Results of assessment and recommendations for treatment. In M.H. Ben-Aron, S.J. Hucker, & C.D. Webster (Eds.), *Clinical criminology: Assessment and treatment of criminal behavior* (pp. 207-220). Toronto: M & M Graphics.

Abel, G.G., Osborn, C.A., & Twigg, D.A. (1993). Sexual assault through the life span. In H. Barbaree, W.L. Marshall, & S.M. Hudson (Eds.). *The juvenile sex offender* (pp. 104-117). New York: The Guilford Press.

Abel, G.G., & Rouleau, J. (1990). The nature and extent of sexual assault. In W.L. Marshall, D.R. Laws, & H.E. Barbaree (Eds.), Handbook of sexual assault: Issues, theories, and treatment of the offender (pp. 9-22). New York: Plenum Press.

Bagley, C., Wood, M., & Young, L. (1994). Victim to abuser: Mental health and behavioral sequels of child sexual abuse in a community survey of young adult males. *Child Abuse and Neglect, 18,* 683-697.

Barbaree, H., Hudson, S.M., & Seto, M.C. (1993). Sexual assault in society: The role of the juvenile offender. In H. Barbaree, W.L. Marshall, & S.M. Hudson (Eds.). *The juvenile sex offender* (pp. 1-24). New York: The Guilford Press.

Becker, J.V., Cunningham-Rathner, J., & Kaplan, M.S. (1986). Adolescent sexual offenders: Demographics, criminal and sexual histories, and recommendations for reducing future offenses. *Journal of Interpersonal Violence, 1,* 431-445.

Becker, J.V., & Kaplan, M.S. (1988). The assessment of adolescent sexual offenders. In R.J. Prinz (Ed.), *Advances in behavioral assessment of children and families* (pp. 97-118). Greenwich, CT: JAI Press.

Bridges, G.S., Conley, D., Beretta, G.R., Engen, R.L., Price-Spratlen, T., Rankin, M., & Steen, S. (1993). *Racial disproportionality in the juvenile justice system: Final report.* Olympia, WA: Washington State Commission on African American Affairs and Management Services Division/Department of Social and Health Services.

Clark, M. (1995, March). *Uniting adolescent sex offenders and their families through treatment.* Keynote Address presented at the National Adolescent Perpetrator Network Meeting, St. Louis, MO.

Davis, G.E., & Leitenberg, H. (1987). Adolescent sex offenders. *Psychological Bulletin, 101,* 417-427.

Federal Bureau of Investigation. (1991). *Uniform crime reports for the United States.* Washington, DC: U.S. Department of Justice.

Federal Bureau of Investigation. (1993). *Uniform crime reports for the United States.* Washington, DC: U.S. Department of Justice.

Fehrenbach, P.A., Smith, W., Monastersky, C., & Deisher, R.W. (1986). Adolescent sexual offenders: Offender and offense characteristics. *American Journal of Orthopsychiatry, 56,* 225-233.

Finkelhor, D., Araji, S., Baron, L., Browne, A., Peters, S.D., & Wyatt, G.E. (1986). *A sourcebook on child sexual abuse.* Newbury Park, CA: Sage Publications.

Ford, M.E., & Linney, J.A. (1995). Comparative analysis of juvenile sexual offenders, violent nonsexual offenders, and status offenders. *Journal of Interpersonal Violence, 10,* 56-70.

Gilby, R., Wolf, L., & Goldberg, B. (1989). Mentally retarded adolescent sex offenders: A survey and pilot study. *Canadian Journal of Psychiatry, 34,* 542-548.

Griffiths, D.M., Quinsey, V.L., & Hingsburger, D. (1989). *Changing inappropriate sexual behavior: A community-based approach for persons with developmental disabilities.* Baltimore: P.H. Brookes Publishing Co.

Huizinga, D., & Elliott, D.S. (1987). Juvenile offenders: Prevalence, offender incidence, and arrest rates by race. *Crime and Delinquency, 33,* 206-223.

Hunter, J.A., Lexier, L.J., Goodwin, D.W., Browne, P.A., & Dennis, C. (1993). Psychosexual, attitudinal, and developmental characteristics of juvenile female sexual perpetrators in a residential treatment setting. *Journal of Child and Family Studies, 2,* 317-326.

Kahn, T.J., & Chambers, H.J. (1991). Assessing reoffense risk with juvenile sexual offenders. *Child Welfare, 70,* 333-345.

Kahn, T.J., & Lafond, M.A. (1988). Treatment of the adolescent sexual offender. *Child and Adolescent Social Work, 5,* 135-148.

Knight, R.A., & Prentky, R. (1993). Exploring characteristics for classifying juvenile sex offenders. In H.E. Barbaree, W.L. Marshall, & S.M. Huson (Eds.), *The juvenile sex offender* (pp. 45-83). New York: The Guilford Press.

Knopp, F.H. (1984). *Remedial intervention in adolescent sex offenses: Nine program descriptions.* Brandon, VT: Safer Society Press.

Knopp, F.H., & Lackey, L.D. (1987). *Female sexual abusers: A summary of data from 44 treatment providers.* Brandon, VT: Safer Society Press.

Krisberg, B., Schwartz, I., Fishman, G., Eisikovits, Z., Guttman, E., & Joe, K. (1987). The incarceration of minority youth. *Crime and Delinquency, 33,* 173-205.

Lane, S. (1991). Sexual abuse cycle. In G.D. Ryan, & S. Lane (Eds.). *Juvenile sexual offending: Causes, consequences, and correction* (pp. 103-142). Lexington, MA: Lexington Books.

McGarrell, E.F. (1993). Trends in racial disproportionality in juvenile court processing: 1985-1989. *Crime and Delinquency, 39,* 29-48.

Marshall, W.L., Laws, D.R., & Barbaree, H.E. (1990). *Handbook of sexual assault: Issues, theories, and treatment of the offender.* New York: Plenum Press.

Mathews, R., Hunter, J.A., & Vuz, J. (1997). Juvenile female sexual offenders: Clinical characteristics and treatment issues. *Sexual Abuse: A Journal of Research and Treatment, 9,* 187-199.

Murphy, W.D., Coleman, E.M., & Haynes, M.R. (1983). Treatment and evaluation issues with the mentally retarded sex offender. In J.G. Greet & I.R. Stuart (Eds.), *The sexual aggressor: Current perspectives on treatment* (pp. 22-41). New York: Van Nostrand Reinhold Co.

National Task Force on Juvenile Sexual Offending. (1993). The revised report from the national task force on juvenile sexual offending 1993, of the national adolescent perpetrator network. *Juvenile and Family Court Journal, 44,* 1-120.

O'Brien, M.J. (1989). *Characteristics of male adolescent sibling incest offenders: Preliminary findings.* Brandon, VT: Safer Society Press.

Rogers, C.M., & Tremaine, T. (1984). Clinical intervention with boy victims of sexual abuse. In S. Greer & I.R. Stuart (Eds.), *Victims of sexual aggression: Men, women, and children* (pp. 91-104). New York: Van Nostrand Reinhold.

Ryan, G.D. (1989). Victim to victimizer: Rethinking victim treatment. *Journal of Interpersonal Violence, 4,* 325-341.

Ryan, G.D., & Lane, S. (1991). Integrating theory and method. In G.D. Ryan, & S. Lane (Eds.). *Juvenile sexual offending: Causes, consequences, and correction* (pp. 255-298). Lexington, MA: Lexington Books.

Ryan, G.D., & Lane, S. (1991). *Juvenile sexual offending: Causes, consequences, and correction.* Lexington, MA: Lexington Books.

Schwartz, I.M. (1989). *(In)justice for juveniles: Rethinking the best interests of the children.* Lexington, MA: Lexington Books.

Showers, J., Farber, E.D., Joseph, J.A., Oshins, L., & Johnson, C.F. (1983). The sexual victimization of boys: A three-year survey. *Health Values: Achieving High-Level Wellness, 7,* 15-18.

Smith, W.R. (1988). Delinquency and abuse among juvenile sexual offenders. *Journal of Interpersonal Violence, 3,* 400-413.

Smith, H., & Israel, E. (1987). Sibling incest: A study of the dynamics of 25 cases. *Child Abuse and Neglect, 11,* 101-108.

Ward, K.M., Heffern, S.J., Wilcox, D.A., McElwee, D., Dowrick, P., Brown, T.D., Jones, M.J., & Johnson, C.L. (1992). *Managing inappropriate sexual behaviors: Supporting individuals with developmental disabilities in the community.* Anchorage, AK: Alaska Specialized Education and Training Services, Inc.

Wasserman, J., & Kappel, S. (1985). *Adolescent sex offenders in Vermont.* Burlington, VT: Vermont Department of Health.

When kids molest kids. *Newsweek,* (1992, March 30) , 68-70.

Worling, J.R. (1995). Adolescent sibling-incest offenders: Differences in family and individual functioning when compared to adolescent nonsibling sex offenders. *Child Abuse and Neglect, 19,* 633-643.

Chapter 2
Cycle of Offense as a Crucial Component of Treatment

The need to identify the components of effective treatment of adolescent sexual offenders in both outpatient and residential settings has been well-documented. The National Task Force on Juvenile Sexual Offending (1993) outlines numerous issues to be addressed in treatment, including:

1. Identification of pattern or cycle of abusive behavior;
2. Interruption of cycle before abusive behavior occurs, and control of abusive behavior;
3. Resolution of victimization in the history of the abusive youth;
4. Development of victim awareness/empathy;
5. Development of internal sense of mastery and control;
6. Understanding the role of sexual arousal;
7. Understanding the consequences of offending behavior for self, the victim, and their families;
8. Identification and remediation, to the extent possible, of family issues or dysfunctions;
9. Identification of cognitive distortions, irrational thinking, or thinking errors that support or trigger offending;
10. Identification and expression of feelings;
12. Development of pro-social relationship skills with peers;
13. Management of addictive/compulsive qualities; and
14. Development of relapse prevention strategies (pp. 43-44).

To maintain continuity and integrity in the therapeutic process, a theory-based framework for treatment is critical (National Task Force on Juvenile Sexual Offending, 1993; Ryan & Lane, 1991; Sermabeikian & Martinez, 1994). Numerous cycles have been outlined in the literature; an entire issue of Interchange (Lane, 1994), the newsletter of the National Adolescent Perpetrator Network, was devoted to various models. Highlighted cycles include Schmerla (undated); Gonzales (1994); O'Conner and Esteve (1994); Turner (1994); Wolf (1994); Ross (1993); Ryan (1993); Ryan (1992); Colorado Domestic Violence Coalition and Colorado Department of Health (1991); Lane (1991); Ryan and Lane (1991); Isaac and Lane (1990); Kahn (1990); Freeman-Longo and Bays (1989); Ryan (1989); Ryan, Lane, Davis and Isaac (1987); Lane and Zamora (1984); and Weissberg (1982). Additionally, a cycle of offense with protection plan detours was outlined in a previous publication (Way & Balthazor, 1990).

The cycle of offense is widely regarded as a clinically useful intervention model, but there is limited empirical evidence of its effectiveness. Only relatively recently has research begun to validate the "steps" within the cycle (Gilgun & Connor, 1990). The cycle's usefulness in treatment and relapse prevention is noted in a small follow-up study by the National Adolescent Perpetrator Network which indicated that youths who had learned to identify and manage their affective "triggers" were less likely to re-offend (Ryan & Miyoshi, 1990). Specifically, Ryan and Myoshi noted that adolescents who did not reoffend during the study time period had learned to identify specific triggers to their offending behavior and had learned how to interrupt their offense cycle (p. 7). This study provides preliminary evidence of specific treatment tasks using the cycle of offense that may help reduce reoffense risk.

Commonalities of Cycles

There are numerous similarities among the twenty or so cycle variations that currently exist. Each evolves from the perspective that an adolescent may progress through a predictable series of steps, decisions, or stages that culminates in offense behavior. Each cycle recognizes that a combination of feelings, thoughts, and behaviors moves the adolescent along the cycle toward the sexually abusive behavior. The various cycles recognize that unique issues in a youth's experience influence his* progression through the cycle. The cycles highlight issues of power and control, dysfunctional defenses, and avoidance. A theme uniting the cycles is the recognition that adolescents make choices, and that sometimes these choices result in victimizing another person.

The intent of these cycles is to help the adolescent understand the progression of behaviors, thoughts, and feelings that lead to the sexual offending behavior. By understanding the cycle of offense, adolescents learn how they moved toward the sexual offense. The explicit and implicit purpose of each cycle variation is to help the adolescent become aware of, and accountable for, his decisions. The cycles also help the adolescent become aware that an offense involves multiple decisions before the decision to molest.

The remainder of this book focuses on a cycle of offense adapted from one detailed by Way and Balthazor (1990). Use of the cycle in individual and group treatment and relapse prevention is outlined.

Cycle of Offense with Recovery Exits

This cycle of offense consists of specific steps in two phases: a smaller, pre-offense, or "everyday" cycle, and a larger, offense-specific cycle (see Figure 2.1).

Note: Because the majority of adolescent offenders in treatment are male, the male pronoun will be used throughout this book. However, as Chapter 1 indicates, female adolescents may also sexually offend and can also benefit from the treatment described here.

Figure 2.1

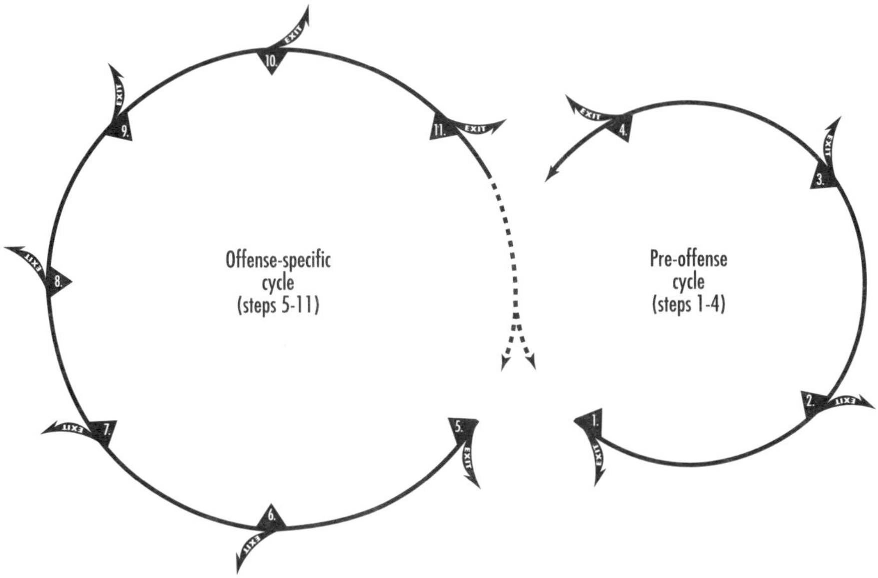

CYCLE OF OFFENSE WITH RECOVERY EXITS

The steps inside the cycle indicate steps the offender may move through that culminate in a sexual offense. The steps outside the cycle indicate the choice points, or exits the offender may use at each step of the cycle to prevent reoffense. Adolescent and adult offenders have provided insight and input on the development of this cycle over the past ten years.

The cycle structures sexual offender treatment and recovery. Its characteristics include:

1. The cycle is broken into two sections, with the first (pre-offense cycle) detailing steps everyone faces in everyday life. The second section (offense cycle) focuses on the steps the adolescent moves through that culminate in a sexual offense (see Figure 2.2);
2. The pre-offense cycle emphasizes the adolescent's commonality with all people and normalizes the difficult decisions made in everyday life;
3. The pre-offense cycle recognizes that an individual's history and core beliefs directly influence daily coping (ATSA, 1997);
4. The offense cycle includes, from the beginning, exits used to prevent relapse;
5. The offense cycle model recognizes that feelings associated with

sexually offending, in and of themselves, further alienate and distance the adolescent from people he is close to;

6. The cycle recognizes, and in fact emphasizes, that to prevent sexual offending behavior, the adolescent must make significant changes early in his cycle before sexual urges occur;
7. Relapse prevention exits are available at each step of the cycle; recognizing that positive choices may be made at any time, thus halting movement toward reoffense;
8. The steps of the cycle and their exits allow the adolescent to learn how his personal decisions culminated in sexually offending and to learn the options he now has to prevent reoffending;
9. The structure of the cycle and relapse prevention exits provide a shorthand way to help an adolescent recognize at any time whether he is in the cycle or in relapse prevention. The exits guide him in preventing relapse.

The following vignette illustrates the use of the cycle in treatment:

> A therapist presented the offense cycle to a mother and grandmother to help them understand their teen's behavior. Afterward, the grandmother said tearfully, "For the first time in my life, I understand why my family has acted the way they have. It seems like our whole family needs help learning how to deal with the divorces and alcoholism we've struggled with." The therapist was then able to use the pre-offense cycle in family therapy to significantly improve the family's communication and relationships. In turn, the teen's support system and aftercare treatment plan were strengthened .*

Most sexual offense cycles focus on the thoughts, feelings, and behaviors of the offender before, during, and after the offense. Though these are essential components of the offense cycle, they are, in fact, manifestations of underlying issues and core beliefs that fuel the cycle and compel the offender to begin or continue in his cycle. It is important to focus on a pre-offense cycle if one is to break the offender's compulsive sequence of thoughts and actions. If these core issues are not addressed and resolved, the adolescent may reoffend or may use other destructive coping attempts such as alcohol or drug abuse, physical or emotional abuse, or other illegal activity to alleviate negative feelings or regain a sense of power and control.

Use of the pre-offense cycle challenges the offender's belief that he is unique as

Note: Case examples have been altered to ensure anonymity.

Figure 2.2

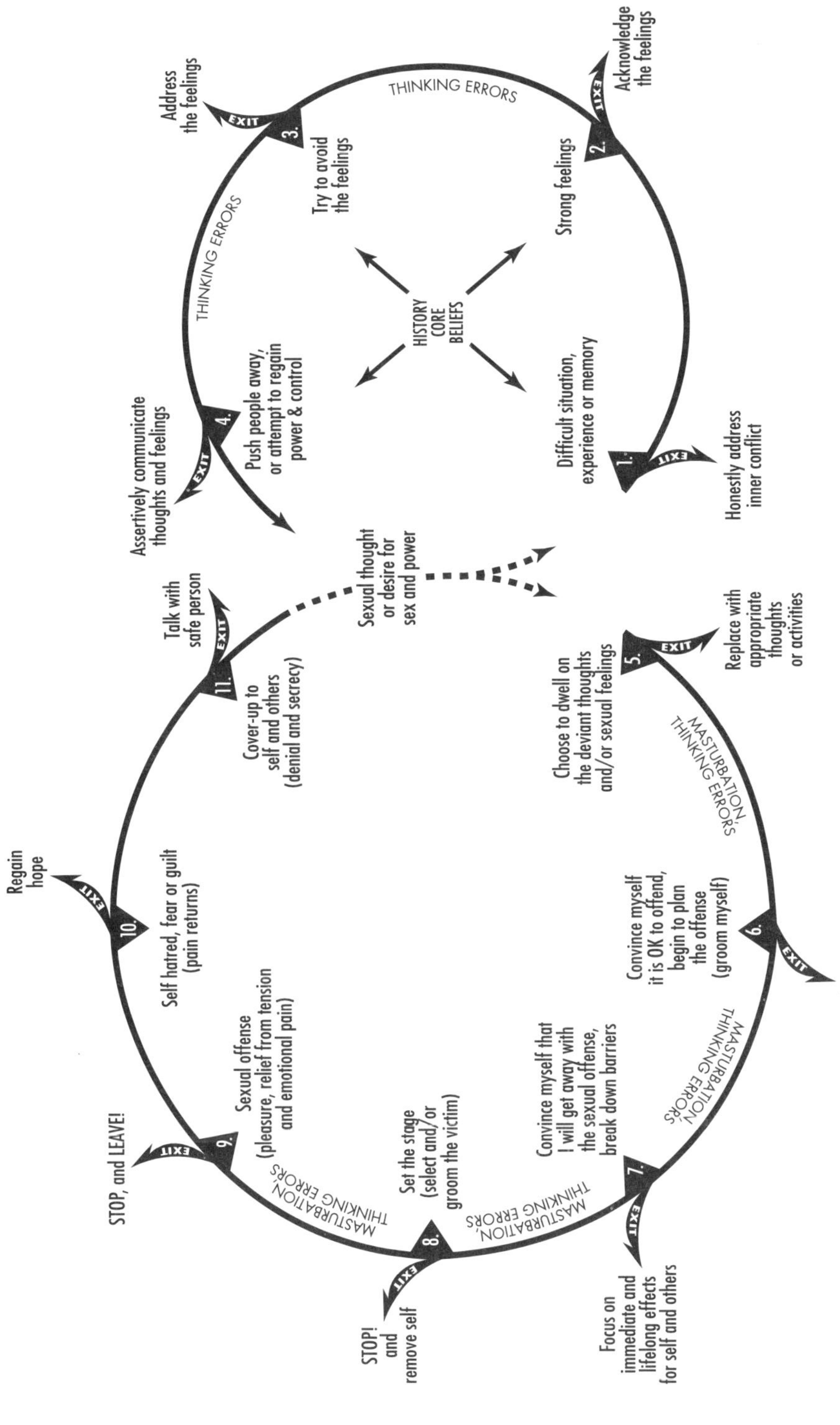

CYCLE OF OFFENSE WITH RECOVERY EXITS

an excuse for his offending behavior. This is accomplished by helping him see that everyone faces difficult situations, experiences, or memories, and that people often have strong feelings regarding those events. The crucial distinction is choosing how to respond, react, and cope with those events and feelings. It is vital for the adolescent to understand that the offense cycle does not begin with a sexual thought or fantasy; rather, it begins much earlier, with ineffective reactions or responses to difficult life experiences.

Using the sexual offense cycle is vital in helping the adolescent address issues and goals in sexual offender treatment, and these include:

1. Explore the etiology, context, and underlying issues of his offending behavior;
2. Clarify the issue of personal responsibility as a therapeutic response to the adolescent's sense that, "It just happened," and emphasize that the decision to molest is the culmination of a process that has many decision points;
3. Identify, confront, and replace the patterns of thoughts and beliefs that led to the adolescent sexually offending against a child;
4. Disclose increasingly in-depth and honest details about his sexual offending behavior;
5. Integrate thoughts, feelings, and behaviors for a comprehensive approach to treatment;
6. Resolve painful memories and difficult issues;
7. Develop an individual relapse prevention plan, thereby responding to the adolescent's statement, "I don't know what else to do";
8. Identify negative patterns of behavior and develop problem-solving and decision-making skills to change these patterns and reduce the adolescent's risk of reoffending;
9. Develop skills for nonexploitive relationships; and
10. Regain trust of family members and significant others.

Once an offender has mastered an understanding of the cycle, the therapist has a tangible framework with which to help the adolescent reach his goals by integrating each goal into one or more steps of the cycle. The following example highlights use of the cycle for multiple tasks:

> One therapist commented, "I've used the cycle a number of times in group. I think it helps adolescents to identify where they are on the cycle and defuses some of the mystery about their offending. Using the cycle seems to clear up those abstract concepts, and introducing the cycle in group has increased interest in using the cycle in individual therapy."

Use of the cycle in treatment is detailed in Chapters 3 and 4 through discussion of the component steps in the cycle and exits for relapse prevention. Before examining the framework of the cycle of offense, it is helpful to understand the larger context of the adolescent's history and core beliefs.

Context for Pre-Offense Cycle

The pre-offense cyclc is a description of the coping processes people face daily. Each of us has the potential to move through these steps as we attempt to reduce or avoid the pain and frustration of difficult situations, experiences, or memories. This struggle may be intensified by sleep deficiency, stress, any difficult situations occurring within a short period, or limited knowledge of healthy coping skills. For adolescent offenders, these negative situations may also include having been sexually or physically abused, growing up with alcoholic parents, or being emotionally abused at an early age. Although the adolescent's reactions may be similar to others', his perceptions of the world and of himself are significantly different; therefore, it is necessary to begin an in-depth examination of sexual offending behavior within the context of these perceptions and reactions.

A cognitive-behavioral framework highlights the connections between physical self, thoughts, feelings, environment, and behavior, and emphasizes that any change, positive or negative, in one area will have consequences (positive or negative) on the others. For example, if physical self, thoughts, feelings, environment, and behavior are represented as a mobile (see diagram), tugging on any one factor will have an immediate and definite impact on the others.

Figure 2.3: Balance of cognitive-behavioral factors

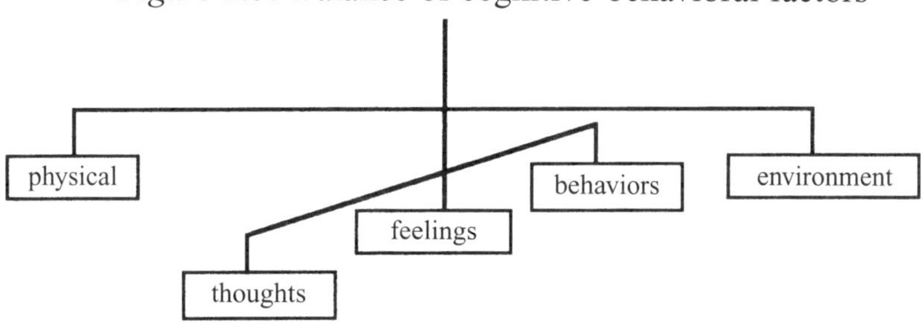

To understand the offender's behavior and his cycle, it is important to examine extreme ways the adolescent may attempt to cope with difficult events and strong unpleasant feelings. He may initially react to and perceive life similarly to others who have experienced a traumatic event. However, as these difficult experiences, situations, or memories are filtered through his core beliefs (beliefs about himself and his relationship to the world), the offender may develop a shame-based thought process that confirms that he is a bad, unworthy, or shameful person and that the world is unsafe or cruel. Alternatively, the adolescent may respond to overwhelming feelings by becoming numb, by assuming the role of victim in his interactions,or by angry retaliation for past events.

As time passes, these thought processes become ingrained and unconscious. Often the offender is unaware that he recites an ongoing monologue as he reacts to the external world. Thoughts such as, "I'll make him do it my way...Why bother...I'm no good...I'll get back at them...I'm always getting picked on...Who cares...They're all against me" are common. This destructive thought pattern adds fuel to the fire of the core beliefs. It is therefore crucial to help the adolescent listen to his inner monologue and begin to evaluate his reactions to various memories and experiences. As the adolescent is able to identify these statements, he can begin to explore the underlying destructive core beliefs and the effect they have on his life. It is important to reiterate that understanding what the adolescent is trying to resolve as the result of his distorted perception or world view is different than excusing the adolescent's offending behavior.

When the therapist and adolescent begin to identify the adolescent's underlying issues and struggles, and connect the sexual behavior with the offender's core beliefs, the adolescent begins to develop a framework to help make sense of a senseless act. As the framework for the cycle of offense is outlined, the offender can retrace his thoughts, feelings, and behaviors to discover the patterns and decisions that led to his offending behavior. To develop this framework, it is helpful for the adolescent to take what he already knows about his environment, physical state, feelings, thoughts, and behaviors and begin to integrate this understanding into Steps 1 through 4 of the cycle (see Table 2.1).

Table 2.1: Comparison of cognitive-behavioral theory and pre-offense cycle steps

Aspects	Steps	Description
Environmental/physical	Step 1	Difficult situation, experience, memory
Feelings	Step 2	Strong feelings
Thoughts	Step 3	Try to avoid the feelings
Behaviors	Step 4	Push people away, or attempt to regain power and control

Once he has developed this framework and explored the impact of his distorted core beliefs, the adolescent can learn to respond to himself and others through healthier and more realistic core beliefs. Later in therapy, the offender learns to recognize warning signs and use exits to intervene in his progression toward offending. It is also important for the offender to filter current difficult situations, experiences, and memories through healthier core beliefs. This allows the offender to begin to break his offense cycle and to function in a different, less destructive manner with others.

Relapse Prevention Plan

A critical aspect of treating adolescent sexual offenders is replacing distorted thinking, dysfunctional attitudes, and destructive behavior patterns with appropriately empowering beliefs, more humane attitudes, and new coping behaviors. Without this difficult but crucial shift, it is difficult to demonstrate to the victim, the victim's family, and the community that this adolescent is less likely to reoffend, and there is no accountability for the treatment program.

It is critical for the adolescent to develop appropriate coping mechanisms to prevent relapse. The following vignette describes one way the cycle is used to accomplish this:

> One treatment facility has used the cycle and relapse prevention plan in all components of its program. Residents use the cycle to explore their behavior and evaluate their motives. The teens frequently talk about which step they are on and what is occurring in their lives. This has also been valuable in ending the typical argument, "Staff always put everything back to sex or my offense. I wasn't acting sexually or even thinking about sex!"

Once adolescents understand the context of their behavior, they are often less defensive in addressing other nonsexual, yet inappropriate or destructive, behaviors.While it may be difficult, if not impossible, to address and resolve all issues before treatment is terminated, it is imperative that the adolescent and members of his support system understand the importance of the entire cycle and the relapse prevention exits. As adolescents progress through treatment and develop more empathy, they may feel shame and self-hatred for the offense they committed. These feelings may convince them that they will not hurt anyone again. At the same time, these new strong feelings of shame and self-loathing ironically may contribute to continued acting out, this time by committing crimes without a visible victim, such as breaking and entering, arson, or destruction of property. The therapist and adolescent must recognize the connection between delinquent behaviors and sexual acting out, as demonstrated by the following example:

> A therapist stated, "I truly believe that Ben will not sexually offend. But

> I am sure that he will continue to be involved in delinquent behavior in the future." The therapist recommended that the adolescent remain in treatment even though he was no longer at high risk to sexually offend.

A structured relapse prevention plan is developed only after the adolescent and therapist have gained an in-depth understanding of the individualized cycle of offending. Relapse prevention can only be accomplished by developing replacement processes. The adage "If you always do what you always did, then you'll always get what you always got" applies here, also. A common statement for adolescents entering treatment is, "I won't ever do this [sexually offend] again." is used to address denial of potential relapse by examining the pre-offense cycle and its relationship to reoffending. It also identifies alternative behaviors and thinking patterns that would more constructively help deter the adolescent from moving through the cycle of offense.

As the adolescent becomes familiar with the protection, or relapse prevention, plan, he must use his new awareness of choices and alternatives to cope with small incidents, difficult situations, uncomfortable experiences, and painful memories in everyday life. In this way, he begins to practice and strengthen new coping patterns that utilize healthy thinking, increase appropriate interactions, and reduce isolation.

References

Association for the Treatment of Sexual Abusers (1997). *Ethical standards and principles for the management of sexual abusers* (2nd ed.). Beaverton, OR: Author.

Gilgun, J.F., & Connor, T.M. (1990). Isolation and the adult male perpetrator of child sexual abuse: Clinical concerns. In A.L. Horton, B.L. Johnson, L.M. Roundy, & D. Williams (Eds.), *The incest perpetrator: A family member no one wants to treat* (pp. 74-87). Newbury Park, CA: Sage Publications.

Knopp, F.H., Freeman-Longo, R., & Stevenson, W.F. (1992). *Nationwide survey of juvenile and adult sexual offender treatment programs and models.* Orwell, VT: The Safer Society Press.

Lane, S. (1994). The cycle. *Interchange, (June),* 1-18.

National Adolescent Perpetrator Network. (1993). The revised report from the national task force on juvenile sexual offending, of the national adolescent perpetrator network. *Juvenile and Family Court Journal. 44,* 1-120.

Ryan, G.D., & Lane, S. (1991). *Juvenile sexual offending: Causes, consequences, and correction.* Lexington, MA: Lexington Books.

Ryan, G.D., & Miyoshi, T. (1990). Summary of a pilot follow-up study of adolescent sexual perpetrators after treatment. *Interchange, (January),* 6-8.

Sermabeikian, P., & Martinez, D. (1994). Treatment of adolescent sexual offenders: Theory-based practice. *Child Abuse and Neglect, 18,* 969-975.

Way, I.F., with Balthazor, T.J. (1990). *Manual for structured group treatment with adolescent sexual offenders.* Notre Dame, IN: Jalice Publishers.

Chapter 3
Steps of the Pre-Offense and Offense Cycles

This chapter discusses the steps of the cycle of offense (see Figure 3.1) and describes how adolescent sexual offenders may move through the steps of the pre-offense and offense cycles to culminate in sexually offending against a child. The steps of the cycle of offense are detailed below:

<u>Pre-offense cycle:</u>

1. Difficult situation, experience, or memory;
2. Strong feelings;
3. Try to avoid the feelings;
4. Push people away, or attempt to regain power and control;

<u>Link between cycles:</u>

Sexual thought or desire for sex and power.

<u>Offense cycle:</u>

5. Choose to dwell on the deviant thoughts and/or sexual feelings;
6. Convince myself it is OK to offend, and begin to plan the offense (groom myself);
7. Convince myself that I will get away with the sexual offense, break down barriers;
8. Set the stage (select and/or groom the victim);
9. Sexual offense (pleasure, relief from tension and emotional pain);
10. Self-hatred, fear or guilt (pain returns);
11. Cover up to self and others (denial and secrecy).

The Pre-Offense Cycle

STEP 1: DIFFICULT SITUATION, EXPERIENCE, OR MEMORY

When someone experiences difficult situations coupled with unhealthy core beliefs, life can appear overwhelming. Examples of difficult situations, experiences, or memories might include a parent's death, parents' divorce, experiencing sexual, physical, verbal or emotional abuse, family'smove to a new home, parent's substance abuse, rejection or abandonment, or harassment by peers.

As the following vignette illustrates, difficult situations can weigh heavily on adolescents:

When Tammy's parents divorced, she was somewhat relieved, yet she felt

Figure 3.1

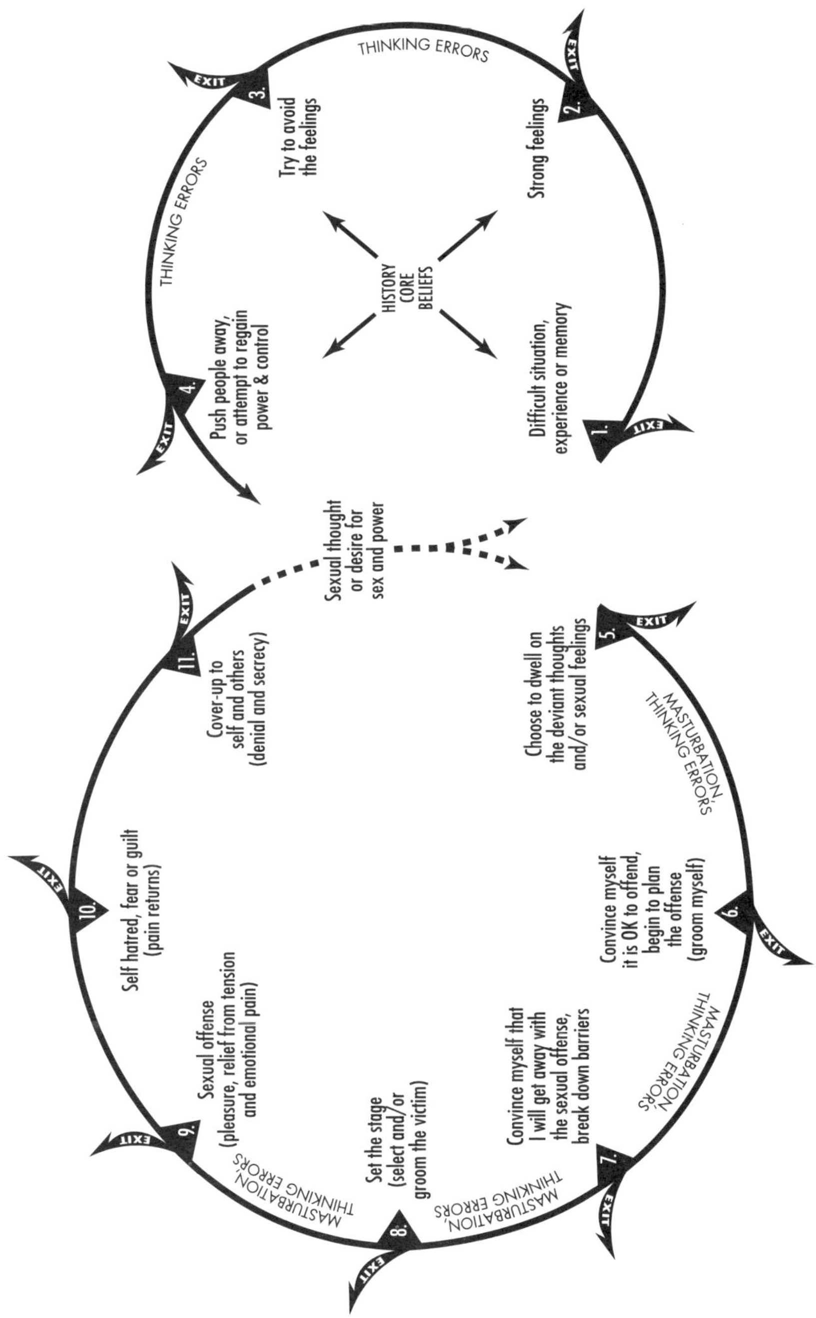

CYCLE OF OFFENSE

> that the divorce was her fault. She thought that if she had been better behaved, her parents might have fought less and therefore would have stayed together. Throughout the marriage, her father was verbally and physically abusive to Tammy and her mother. Tammy remembers her father verbally degrading her and making her feel worthless. When he left, her mother became depressed and began to drink alcohol on a daily basis.

In many families, difficult situations are often managed by using unproductive coping mechanisms. Within this context, children begin to develop an understanding of their world and learn how to interact with it. As in Tammy's family, when dysfunctional coping strategies such as denial, repression, projection, avoidance, and substance abuse are used frequently, children typically do not learn how to cope directly with difficulty. If children respond to difficulties using the flawed coping skills they have learned at home, they are met with resistance and disapproval from those outside their families, thus confirming their sense that the world is unsafe, antagonistic, and untrustworthy. Parents may reinforce this belief by reminding the child to be fearful of strangers and emphasizing that what happens in the family must be kept within the family. As children carry these dysfunctional core beliefs into adolescence, they are unprepared and unskilled for addressing or overcoming difficulties.

STEP 2: STRONG FEELINGS

As with all of us, adolescents react to difficult situations, experiences, or memories with strong feelings. These may include anger, grief and loss, sadness, depression, powerlessness, helplessness, rejection, abandonment, fear, discouragement, frustration, hopelessness, rage, or despair. These feelings may be overwhelming.

The following vignette demonstrates how normal feelings may also be discounted by others:

> Jimmy had fallen on a trampoline and his arm was noticeably broken. As he came up to his father crying and holding out his arm, his father angrily shushed Jimmy, saying, "What are you crying for now, you wuss...You're always crying about something!" Jimmy immediately became quiet, withdrawn, and stopped crying.

These strong feelings are in direct correlation to the adolescent's beliefs and perceptions of himself and the world around him. Often these feelings become threatening through their own "unleashed" power and strength. This is especially true for the adolescent whose feelings remind him of past experiences where he felt stripped of his control and dignity; therefore, the experience can be increasingly painful as the feelings create a chain reaction to other strong feelings that the adolescent is unable to resolve.

Strong feelings may be associated with such healthy desires as the need for love, intimacy, nurturing, and acceptance; however, if the adolescent feels that it is impossible to satisfy or meet these needs, the pain he believes the needs create becomes more intense. For adolescents who were socialized to be strong, independent, self-sufficient, and capable, these needs are not experienced or perceived as acceptable. Others who were abandoned, abused, or neglected may have difficulty believing their needs for love and nurturing will ever be met.

Because these feelings and needs persist but are perceived as socially and psychologically inappropriate or overwhelming, adolescents are faced with a dilemma. They are unable to make situations disappear, and the painful feelings threaten their psychological equilibrium; yet life must go on. This in turn magnifies the situation, experience, or memory, and leaves the adolescent feeling out of control. Because the world appears antagonistic, adolescents begin to turn inward and develop an internal "reality" that is safer, more pleasant, and seemingly invincible. In doing so, they attempt to avoid all negative feelings and/or begin to look for ways to regain control.

STEP 3: TRY TO AVOID THE FEELINGS

Americans spend millions of dollars a year in an attempt to escape reality or numb emotional pain, including the use of legal and illegal drugs. Advertisers invest extensive amounts of time and money to persuade people that bigger boats, fancier cars, cosmetic makeovers, and other products and services will satisfy unmet needs. Sexuality is often used to sell products. For the adolescent offender, this message is not only appealing but can be used to justify his core belief that "sex is my most important need and is the only way to make me feel good or to get power and control."

Many offenders try to avoid the pain of negative feelings. Many have spent much of their lives avoiding the painful emotions connected to trauma-based experiences. As the emotions are sidestepped, the adolescent becomes convinced that this is the only way to survive. This denial of his own feelings subsequently blinds him to the pain of the children he molests. This avoidance may also take the form of dissociation, as detailed in the following vignette:

> Samuel was molested from ages 3 to 8 by his stepfather. He pushed these thoughts and feelings to the back of his mind so often and repetitively that they became buried. At age 8 he began to sexually abuse children

> who were much younger than himself over a period of one year. He then repressed his memory of the sexual offense behavior and began setting fires and other delinquent behaviors. Later, when confronted with the original police report, Samuel began crying and stated, "I can't believe I did that, but it must be true...I hate myself."

Some adolescents experience a strong desire to regain a sense of control and power in order to prevent themselves from drowning in their own "sea of feelings." This avoidance is fueled by distorted thinking, such as, "A real man would be able to handle this...These feelings are not cool...I can't deal with feeling this way...This is too scary...I'll go crazy if I feel this way much longer...I must be crazy...I hate this, but there is nothing that I can do to change it."

For children raised in dysfunctional or multi-problem families, ineffective and inappropriate coping skills become ingrained. This often occurs simply because the problem, like the proverbial elephant in the living room, is ignored. The adolescent observes family members investing all of their energy in pretending or refusing to see that a problem exists, either indirectly or blatantly. Although the adolescent may initially acknowledge the absurdity of the family's reaction, he begins to see their coping mechanisms as "the norm," and learns that avoidance is the safest way to handle problems.

> Edward stated that it was easier to live in his fantasy world where he was in control than to live in reality where his parents and friends were mean and rejecting. He continued, "Life hurts too much, and I'm sick of being hurt!"

A primary form of avoidance is through such behaviors as finding another activity, walking away from the situation, playing video or computer games, listening to music, purposely thinking about something or someone else, watching television or a movie, or reading a magazine, all of which also can be healthy, self-reinforcing distractions. Problems may develop, however, when such distractions are used to pretend that the difficult situation, feeling, or experience does not exist, or to avoid it entirely. The adolescent also avoids feelings through self-talk such as, "I don't care...It doesn't bother me...No one cares...So what...I can handle this alone."

An example of a day on the beach is instructive. It is difficult to hold an inflated beach ball underwater. Yet, with determination, energy, and focus, it can be done; however, it is impossible to do anything else at the same time. In the same way, the adolescent can succeed at avoiding the strong, unwanted feelings. He will often suppress them and tell himself that they do not exist; however, he cannot at the same time pursue meaningful relationships or personal growth. This is critical because the need to be liked and accepted is vital for adolescents. In the same way that the adolescent learns to avoid his own painful feelings, he also develops a denial of the pain of others, which provides a context for objectifying the child he sexually victimizes. The following vignette demonstrates this attempt to avoid feelings:

> When John talked about his painful relationship with his father, he often said, "It doesn't matter," or, "I don't care anymore." As he tried to ignore his painful feelings, he maintained that things were more important than people. John would often state that he only kept his father in his life "to get money or things". However, no matter how hard John tried, there were times when he reluctantly admitted that he did care about his father and that he was hurt by his father's apparent rejection. This disclosure would then anger John as he realized that he had failed to convince himself that he did not care, and that he had failed in being "good enough" to gain his father's approval.

Just as the beach ball held underwater fights to resurface, repressed feelings also fight to resurface, especially at difficult times, thus reminding the adolescent that denying them is nearly impossible. Therefore, strong feelings become a pursuing enemy that the adolescent cannot totally avoid.

STEP 4: PUSH PEOPLE AWAY, OR ATTEMPT TO REGAIN POWER AND CONTROL

Due to beliefs such as, "No one will love me as I am," and, "If I let someone come close, he will abuse or have power over me," the adolescent strengthens his belief that his needs will never be met if he has to depend on others. Although the adolescent, like all people, has a basic need to be nurtured and cared for, the fear of rejection and abandonment becomes overwhelming. Thus, he learns to isolate himself, and learns to avoid intimacy and vulnerability at all costs.

Protective self-talk used by the adolescent includes, "Hey, this is working well...I feel better when I don't deal with this problem (in fact, I don't even really have a problem)...Who needs anyone else?...I can take care of myself...No one can even tell that something's wrong...No one really cares anyway." These self-talk statements are examples of cognitive distortions, or "thinking errors." A thinking error is "an undercurrent of misinformation, strange beliefs, myths and/or attitudes which lead to decisions based on faulty perceptions" (Lakey, 1995). When energy is invested in an attempt to deny "the elephant in the room," others who may want to talk about the issue or ask questions become a threat to the fragile avoidance system.

Lakey (1995) identifies a number of thinking errors used by adolescents who sexually offend, including:

1. Making excuses, blaming others, assuming the victim stance when asked to be accountable ("If Mom hadn't let my sister run around with no clothes, I wouldn't be in placement");
2. Feeling superior and above the law ("Those rules don't apply to me because I can do whatever I want; besides, I thought I wouldn't get caught");
3. Not considering, or simply ignoring, how one's behavior might affect others ("I was molested, so I wanted to pass on the pain I felt, and I thought that would make me feel better");
4. Being chronically angry, especially when one cannot gain power and control ("Real men are supposed to intimidate others by acting angry; that's the way they control their women");
5. Expecting others to fall into line with one's own desires and emphasizing one's own uniqueness as a justification for that expectation ("The world - parents, siblings, peers, etc. - owes me because I am so superior and different");
6. Being in touch with reality but not thinking realistically about life; constantly scheming to beat the system ("My judge made a mistake in placing me here. All I have to do is write him, and he'll send me home").

Lane (1991) groups thinking errors into categories of victim stance, negative anticipation, hopelessness, blaming others, control seeking, and justification, and suggests that the adolescent uses different distortions at various points in the cycle (p. 115).

The adolescent may believe that he is the only person experiencing these unpleasant feelings and may be afraid to share them with others. This powerful sense of being alone in the world can become overwhelming and all-consuming. Although he may desire to talk to someone about various feelings and actions, he is unable to trust and has convinced himself that "I don't want to be weak in front of others," or, "If I tell someone how I feel, they won't understand."

At this point, the adolescent will do whatever he believes is necessary to avoid meaningful contact with anyone who might disrupt his avoidance system. Intimacy and vulnerability are avoided through any behavior, attitude, or pattern of interaction that keeps others at a distance.

Some adolescents may avoid their painful reality by channeling their energy into seeking high marks in school, "looking good," participating in special activities or events, becoming involved in social causes, etc., all the while maintaining an emotional distance from those around them. Other adolescents revert to distancing behaviors such as verbal abuse, fighting, using obscenities, isolating, abusing alcohol or drugs, antagonizing, being sarcastic, skipping school, seeking revenge, refusing to engage in conversation, using oppositional behavior, or in general rejecting others before they can be rejected. Regardless of which distancing behavior is selected, the adolescent attempts to regain a sense of power and control over himself and his world while avoiding intimacy. The following vignette highlights the adolescent's irrational belief that one way to avoid pain is to inflict it on others:

> Billie was severely sexually and physically abused by his father from ages two to seven. Initially, Billie would scream, begging his mother to make him stop; however, his mother would not intervene. As the abuse intensified, his mother also molested Billie. When the abuse was reported and Billie was removed from the home, he refused to allow anyone to become emotionally close to him. He told his therapist that his goal in life was to hurt as many people as possible.

At this stage of the cycle, the adolescent becomes isolated from people in his immediate world who can help. A complex interaction of feelings, attitudes, thoughts, and beliefs walls the adolescent off from interactions with people. He refuses or is unable to accept the help he desires; yet, he is dissatisfied with the loneliness. The adolescent believes he must regain control over the situation any way he can. The following vignette details this attempt to regain control:

> Before his parents' divorce, Jason's father sexually abused him. His mother's stated reason for divorcing her husband was that she did not want to live with a "faggot." Jason believed that his mother hated his father for being a "faggot," and she must also hate him for having been sexual with his father. Jason became resentful of his mother's close relationship with his sister. He stated, "I knew I could get back at my mother by sexually hurting my sister. If I was going to be a bad kid, so was she."

Thus, the first four steps of the cycle portray an intense internal struggle. Pain has become an enemy. The fear of rejection is in direct conflict with the need for nurturing. The fear of being overpowered or consumed outweighs the desire for emotional intimacy with another person; therefore, the need to maintain power and control over himself and others becomes a driving force for the adolescent.

The Offense Cycle

At the juncture of the pre-offense and offense cycles, the adolescent has a sexual thought or desire for sex and power. This may occur by seeing something sexual in the media, having a memory or flashback, seeing or meeting someone, experiencing a spontaneous sexual urge, or misinterpreting a nonsexual event - for example, a child sitting on his lap. The initial arousal, in and of itself, is not a choice; however, once the arousal occurs, a conscious decision must be made about a response. The sexual thought combined with the thought or need for power and/or control is a significant experience for the adolescent. What distinguishes the offender from others is how he chooses to respond to that sexual thought.

STEP 5: CHOOSE TO DWELL ON THE DEVIANT THOUGHTS AND/OR SEXUAL FEELINGS

The adolescent progresses in the cycle as he dwells on a sexual thought. As he focuses on the thought, nurtures it, cultivates it, and brings it purposefully to mind when it is absent, the thought becomes more entrenched. The sexual feeling alone can be so attractive and exciting to the offender that he begins to create and live in a fantasy world that is "free" of the stressors that he experienced in the pre-offense cycle. The following vignette demonstrates the power of such thoughts:

> John recalled a time when he was in elementary school and saw a naked older man in the locker room at the community pool. John had never seen an adult's penis before and was confused and excited by what he saw. When John got home, he began to think about this man and wished that he could see a penis again; however, John was scared that his peers would make fun of him if he told them how he felt. As John's thoughts progressed, he began to think about what the penises of younger boys would look like.

When people dwell on sexual fantasies, they often become aroused and some may masturbate to the thought. When the process of dwelling on the thought is accompanied by masturbation, the thought process becomes reinforced by the pleasure and intensity of masturbation; when the thoughts are of an abusive nature, the risk of abusive behavior increases. It is recognized that sexual offenders often use deviant masturbation fantasies to rehearse their sexual offense. Lane (1991) describes a progression of fantasies, from "control-based retaliatory thoughts, to sexual thoughts that involve some element of control, then to contemplation of sexually abusive behaviors" (p. 127). Accompanying thinking errors may include, "I'm not hurting anyone...Everyone masturbates...I have to get rid of this thought somehow...It helps relax me." This pattern may become compulsive and can occur frequently throughout the day as a way to avoid painful issues; however, the relief is temporary. For many adolescent offenders, once they have reached orgasm, their self-hatred, shame, or guilt returns, thus confirming their belief that they are basically bad, unworthy, and unable to control themselves. Alternatively, adolescents may have no guilt nor recognition that this pattern is problematic.

Interestingly, some offenders who refrain from masturbation develop thinking errors to irrationally justify having sex with a young child. Examples of these thinking errors include, "There's nothing wrong with sex with a child as long as he doesn't say no...It's better to have sex with a kid than to play with myself."

STEP 6: CONVINCE MYSELF IT IS OK TO OFFEND, BEGIN TO PLAN THE OFFENSE (GROOM MYSELF)

With this step, the sexual thought moves from a fantasy into a possibility. The act is minimized, justified, rationalized, defended, and normalized through a process of thoughts, attitudes, and beliefs. The adolescent then convinces himself that his sexual activity would be justified, if not deserved. The negative and painful effects that the perpetration would have on the victim are disregarded. Thinking errors may include, "He likes me...It didn't hurt when it happened to me...As long as she is sleeping she won't know or remember...He is too young to know or care...She deserves it...It would be good for him to learn about sex...I bet she would like it." An offender may also use such thinking errors as, "I can stop at any time...She wants this as much as I do...I'll just touch him...I love her and she's the only person who loves me." The offender may also pretend that the sibling is a peer or same-age girlfriend. As the offender continues to fantasize, these thinking errors are reinforced.

As these desires for power and control become linked with sexual thoughts and feelings, the adolescent offender may convince himself that he has the right to take out his anger by sexually assaulting someone. The desire to dominate or be sexual with someone arises from distorted thinking about sexuality, as the following vignette illustrates:

> After his parents divorced, Jason was angry at his father for molesting him and at his mother for treating him "like dirt". He also resented his sister for not being abused, and wished he was a girl. As his hatred grew, Jason decided that it was "OK" to abuse his sister and thought, "It will also be a way to prove that I'm not gay...and, if I am dirt, then what difference does it make what I do anyway?"

Once the offender has distanced himself from his own painful feelings, he becomes unable and/or unwilling to think about what others may think or feel. As he plans his offense and convinces himself that his actions are justified, he grooms himself. He may also project thoughts and feelings onto a potential victim and believe that this child desires to be sexual with him, as in the following example:

> Doug often went to the playground with his younger sister. As he watched his sister and her friends play, he fantasized about being sexual with them. Each time a child looked at him or asked him to play, he convinced himself that the child wanted to be sexual with him.

During treatment many adolescents are amazed to recognize how they groomed themselves to believe it would be all right to offend a child. The following vignette demonstrates:

> When Anthony began to learn about his cycle in treatment, he stated that he now realized how he had convinced himself to initiate the sexual offense against his sister. Anthony reported that he was sexually involved with his girlfriend when he was 12. When she moved away, he became more and more frustrated with the thought of not having a sexual relationship. He stated that he then groomed himself to believe it would be OK for him to molest his eight year-old sister by telling himself, "It will only happen once or twice until I find another girlfriend."

While fantasizing, the offender may act out parts of his fantasy, or imagine that the child is in the room with him. This active fantasy is used to self-medicate. While the adolescent fantasizes, he is able to block out pain, frustration, and boredom. The adolescent thus reconfirms that sex and/or power are better than his present situation; however, when the fantasy by itself becomes unsatisfactory, he begins to think about how to act it out.

STEP 7: CONVINCE MYSELF THAT I WILL GET AWAY WITH THE SEXUAL OFFENSE, BREAK DOWN BARRIERS

Because a small part of the adolescent continues to believe that it really is wrong to sexually offend, he must convince himself that he could get away with the perpetration. The sexual offender intensifies his plan and begins to break down normal social barriers such as moral and ethical taboos, the threat of incarceration and public disgrace, and the fear of getting caught. The possibility of the offense becomes an active plan, and the offender begins to rationalize potential opportunities and possible victims, using such thinking errors as, "She's too young to talk...He'll sleep through it...I could threaten him...If I pick that shy kid, she won't tell." This "superman" thinking is used by the adolescent to continue advancing in the cycle. Some offenders may replay an offense fantasy while thinking of ways to keep from getting caught. Other offenders may move through this step more impulsively.

STEP 8: SET THE STAGE (SELECT AND/OR GROOM THE VICTIM)

Oncc an offender has convinced himself that he will get away with the sexual offense, he begins to set the stage by grooming the child or adult victim. Alternatively, he may prepare himself to molest through other such paraphilic behaviors as voyeurism and exhibitionism. He actively seeks opportunities and environments that would give him access to children. He may offer to baby-sit, frequent video arcades or parks, befriend a child or family, spend time with his siblings, or scout out secluded areas. The following vignette illustrates:

> After looking through his father's pornography, Sandy began to think about how he could see his sister naked. He knew his parents regularly left them alone evenings when they played cards at a neighbor's home. As he thought about the possibility, he became sexually aroused.

An offender may groom his victim in various ways, including developing trust and a false sense of intimacy; threatening the child; initiating horseplay; testing the child's willingness to keep secrets; gradually introducing sexual conversations and stimuli; using manipulation; using physical force, intimidation, or bribery; establishing a relationship; or choosing infants or young children who do not have the cognitive or emotional maturity to know that sexual abuse is wrong. Depending on the grooming technique, this stage may pass quickly or may take months to complete, as detailed in the following vignette:

> Tony spent months grooming his two younger male cousins. He built a clubhouse and invited them to join. Initially, they spent time exploring the woods and coming up with rules for their club. Tony began to implement rules and activities that were more daring. He realized he could hold this against them if they decided to tell others any "secrets." With each step, Tony looked for opportunities to become sexual with his cousins.

Although the adolescent has not yet perpetrated at this point in the cycle, it is often the adolescent offender's attraction to risk that provides the adrenaline rush that becomes self-reinforcing. This focus on self and satisfying self without regard to others allows the adolescent to remain in his narcissistic, distorted world. Many adolescents continue to masturbate throughout the steps of the offense cycle, which reinforces their thinking errors and intensifies their sexual feelings.

STEP 9: SEXUAL OFFENSE (PLEASURE, RELIEF FROM TENSION AND EMOTIONAL PAIN)

Without intervention, the cycle of thoughts, feelings, and behaviors culminates in the adolescent sexually offending against a child, peer, or adult. While sexually offending, the offender focuses only on himself, rather than on his victim. Other people become sexual objects, and the offender uses them to gratify his own needs and desires. Many offenders block out the other person and later are unable to describe the child's face or the child's reaction to the sexual abuse. Thoughts of the effects of the abuse on the other person are either nonexistent or are rationalized, and the focus is primarily on the pleasure and/or power the offense provides the perpetrator. The following example illustrates:

> When Tony thought he had enough to hold over his cousins, he introduced pornography and masturbation into the club. He told them that all older guys "jerk off," and it was a normal way to learn about sex. He then included games that were progressively more deviant and degrading. Tony later admitted that once he stepped into the clubhouse, the rest of the world seemed to disappear, and his two cousins were no longer his cousins, but bodies to experiment with and manipulate for his own sexual gratification.

A critical aspect of the offense cycle is that at the moment of the sexual offense the offender experiences temporary relief from the psychic pain triggered at the beginning of the cycle. This relief becomes powerfully self-reinforcing, and provides the ultimate escape for psychic pain.

STEP 10: SELF HATRED, FEAR, OR GUILT (PAIN RETURNS)

Once the offense is completed, the offender's distortions quickly lose their strength. The thought of getting caught or the reality of the sexual act may overwhelm the offender. The initial pleasure, relief, and sense of power are short-lived, and some offenders begin to regret their actions; yet the memory of the sexual pleasure and escape from painful reality lingers.

It should be noted that some youth use antisocial thoughts to convince themselves that the sexual act itself is not an offense. The belief is that the only wrong is getting caught; therefore, there is no perceived guilt or shame, and the adolescent returns to the act again and again. Alternatively, some adolescents may experience the risk of getting caught as part of the thrill. The power associated with successfully avoiding detection is a secondary reinforcement.

Some adolescents reoffend even though the shame, fear, and/or guilt are overwhelming. In their minds, sexually offending someone is the only thing that eases the pain; however, the offense confirms their inadequacy, ugliness, and difference from the rest of the world. The offense also confirms the adolescent's core belief that he is bad and unworthy. He is convinced that no one could, or would, love him for who he really is; therefore, he remains isolated, fearing that someone will discover the truth.

STEP 11: COVER-UP TO SELF AND OTHERS (DENIAL AND SECRECY)

Although the adolescent has convinced himself at one level that his actions are justified, it is interesting to note that on another level, he does everything in his power to make sure that he is not caught. For many offenders the fear of getting caught is intense. They will utilize any means available to keep the victim quiet and available for further sexual gratification, including physical threats or abuse, intimidation, or bribery. The approach is usually correlated with the manner in which he chose to offend (for example, if he used bribery to coerce the victim, he may continue to use bribery afterward). At this point, the grooming pattern is refined further. Alternatively, the adolescent may do nothing and then have to cope with the fear of getting caught. Other offenders who are intensely self-gratifying may move on immediately after the offense without reflecting at all on the sexual assault or experiencing embarrassment or shame.

As the offender copes with the offense he has committed, it frequently becomes the new difficult situation that places him once more at the beginning of the pre-offense cycle. This presents another situation with which to cope. Other adolescents may skip early steps of the cycle and move immediately to Step 8 (Set the stage - select and groom victim), and set up the next offense; thus, the adolescent continues in the cycle of offense. In this way, the adolescent moves through the pre-offense cycle (ineffective coping and thinking errors) and through the offense cycle (deviant sexual thoughts, grooming both himself and potential victims, planning the sexual offense, committing it, and coping ineffectively with the consequences). This cycle then becomes more ingrained with each offense.

Not all adolescents progress through the steps of the cycle exactly as outlined in this chapter; therefore, it is important to help them understand their individualized cycle steps in treatment. The highly compulsive individual develops a closed cycle and sexual offending behavior takes on a life of its own; his whole day can be one long urge. These adolescents do not identify discreet urges; their daylong focus is on creating the opportunity to offend. One must recognize that for some adolescents, the steps of the cycle are clearly defined; others skip steps or move quickly through them. Some individuals are purely peer-influenced and have not participated in a grooming process. See Appendices C and D for further detail on typology variations for male and female sexual offenders (Mathews, 1994; O'Brien & Bera, 1986; see also, Mathews, Hunter, & Vuz, 1997). It is important that the | adolescent fully disclose his pattern of offending so he can recognize his own progression through the offense cycle. A variety of assessment tools (polygraph, questionnaires, verbal sexual history, sexual lifeline, collateral interviews, etc.) may be used to obtain this information, as illustrated in the following vignette:

> Nick, age 16, attempted to, and seduced, some caregivers (foster parents, mental health practitioners) a number of times. In his lifeline, he disclosed that he had been molested at age 5 by his teenage sister and her friends. Prominent in his memory was their laughter and giggling at his genitals. Through the lifeline, he began to understand that his sexual assaults were an attempt to gain mastery over that experience.

It is crucial for adolescents to thoroughly understand their own individual cycle of offense if they are to engage in the critical task of developing and implementing their personal relapse prevention plan.

References

Lakey, J.F. (1995). Thinking errors in adolescent sex offenders. *Treatment Today,* p. 31.

Lane, S. (1991). The sexual abuse cycle. In G.D. Ryan & S.L. Lane (Eds.), *Juvenile sexual offending: Causes, consequences, and correction* (pp. 103-141). Lexington, MA: Lexington Books.

Mathews, R. (1994). Preliminary adolescent female sexual offender typology. In T. Connor, M. Frost, R. Mathews, J. Raymaker, & S. Wolsleger (Eds.), *Adolescent female sexual offenders: A descriptive and comparative study and treatment manual.* Report #SP-93-0053. St. Paul, MN: The St. Paul Foundation..

Mathews, R., Hunter, J.A., & Vuz, J. (1997). Juvenile female sexual offenders: Clinical characteristics and treatment issues. *Sexual Abuse: A Journal of Research and Treatment, 9,* 187-199.

O'Brien, M., & Bera, W. (1986). Adolescent sexual offenders: A descriptive typology. *Preventing Sexual Abuse, 1,* 1-4.

Chapter 4

Relapse Prevention Exits

Relapse prevention that protects further victimization of children is the primary goal of intervention with adolescent sexual offenders. Certainly, an effective response by the criminal justice system to the sexual offender provides a powerful foundation for relapse prevention when adolescents recognize that they will be held accountable for their criminal behavior. Parents who contact law enforcement officials rather than attempting to handle the problem themselves also play a major role. When this systemic response also includes knowledgeable treatment providers who integrate treatment and relapse prevention, the risk of reoffense is further reduced.

Once an adolescent has begun therapy, the treatment provider has an ethical and professional responsibility to the child who was sexually abused, the community, the offender's family, the offender, and the referring agency. This includes demonstrating that treatment is effective and meaningful in providing the adolescent an opportunity to reduce his risk of reoffense. To accomplish this, the adolescent must develop an individualized relapse prevention plan and integrate it daily into each part of his life. One barrier to this is the offender's strong tendency to compartmentalize his feelings, thoughts, and behaviors. He may demonstrate this by utilizing the relapse prevention plan only during treatment sessions, while resorting to familiar, but flawed, patterns of power and control in interactions with others, as the following vignette highlights:

> During group sessions, Bob appropriately challenged other members when they attempted to overpower a peer or made demeaning comments, and he took responsibility for his behavior when he was confronted. Outside of group, however, Bob perpetuated power struggles with both peers and staff. When confronted, he stated, "We're not in group now, so what's the big deal?"

Effective relapse prevention begins by examining in detail the adolescent's ineffective coping response at each step of the pre-offense cycle, identifying his thinking errors, and detailing alternatives at each step. This is best accomplished by examining the adolescent's daily interactions from a perspective that focuses on relapse prevention in the pre-offense cycle. The following vignette demonstrates:

> After the therapist greeted Darryl in the waiting room, he "power-gripped" her hand in response to her handshake. When the therapist told him that this was painful, he laughed, pointed to his mother, and replied,

"She did it." Darryl was confronted in the session about how his denial of responsibility for his behavior and his inability to acknowledge the pain of the therapist was similar to blaming his sister for "wanting" the sexual abuse, and ignoring her feelings and reactions. As the session progressed, he was able to examine his cycle of offense and relapse prevention accountability in relation to that day's incident and to his sexual abuse of his sister.

This chapter examines relapse prevention by detailing each offense cycle step, identifying the relapse prevention exit for that step, and outlining the changes in beliefs, attitudes, and behaviors the adolescent needs to accomplish (see Figure 4.1). The exit titles are presented as broad guides to assist adolescents in individualizing an effective relapse prevention plan. It is critical for an offender to examine in-depth his grooming process and how he set up his offenses if he is to fully integrate specific individualized exits that are meaningful for him and realistic to maintain on a daily basis. Relapse prevention must become an accepted way of life for him.

The relapse prevention exits include:

Pre-offense cycle

1. Honestly address inner conflict;
2. Acknowledge the feelings;
3. Address the feelings;
4. Assertively communicate thoughts and feelings.

Offense cycle

5. Replace with appropriate thoughts or activities;
6. See the person, and strengthen the barriers;
7. Focus on immediate and lifelong effects for self and others;
8. STOP! and remove self;
9. STOP, and LEAVE!;
10. Regain hope;
11. Talk with safe person.

STEP 1 - Difficult situation, experience, or memory
EXIT 1: HONESTLY ADDRESS INNER CONFLICT

Because all of us face difficult situations, experiences, or memories, we all must learn to honestly address inner conflicts and resolve these situations. When a youth has had extensive life experiences that reinforce his abusive beliefs, therapy must

Figure 4.1

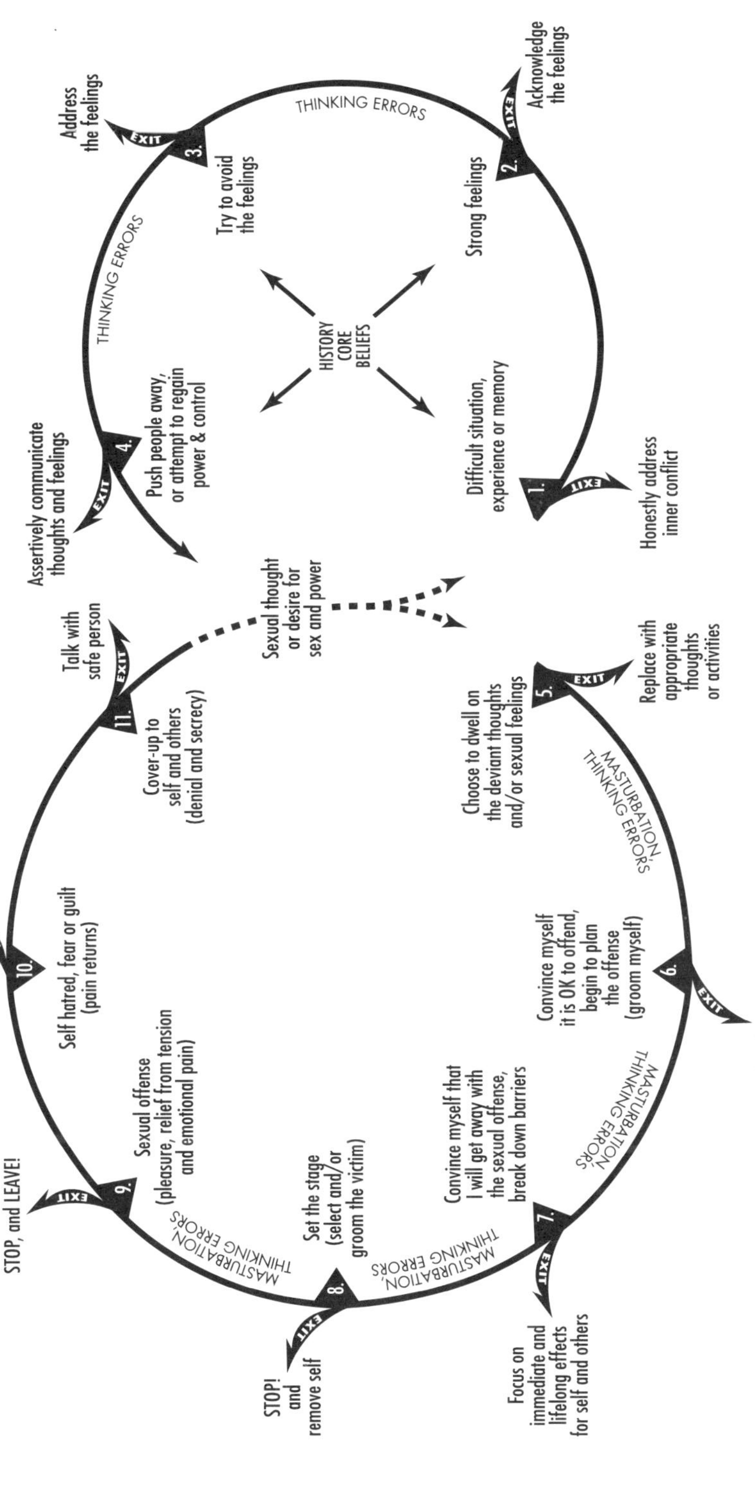

CYCLE OF OFFENSE WITH RECOVERY EXITS

afford him a new experience before the beliefs can be re-framed as no longer being rational. This process takes time but is critical in providing a realistic basis for the youth to change core beliefs about the world and about relationships. The following vignette illustrates:

> Stan was sexually abused by a baby sitter and again by a neighbor boy. He questioned whether it was his fault. His mother told him, "The past is the past and we don't talk about it"; thus, Stan continued to believe that the abuse was his fault. Once Stan understood the importance of exploring and talking about difficult situations, memories, and experiences, he was able to discuss with his therapist the sexual abuse he had experienced. With the help of the therapist, Stan then explored how his own victimization had affected his core beliefs and his relationships with others.

Exits at this step are best learned by processing everyday occurrences as illustrated in the following vignette:

> When Darryl was assisted in talking about what was going on for him when he power-gripped the therapist's hand, he acknowledged that because he had disclosed a lot in the previous session he didn't want to be at the therapy session that day. He said he had gotten scared the previous week about how honest he had been. The therapist acknowledged the difficulty of beginning to break rules about secrecy and they processed how rules for honesty in the session were different from the unstated rules for avoiding direct communication in his family.

This vignette also emphasizes the need to work with the family system so that when the adolescent is helped to make changes, the family is also assisted in identifying and changing problematic communication patterns. Chapter 6 discusses how to share the cycle with parents and family members.

STEP 2 - Strong feelings
EXIT 2: ACKNOWLEDGE THE FEELINGS

Because of the complexity and intensity of the adolescent's feelings and his inability to recognize and normalize those that are related to vulnerability and powerlessness, he must learn to identify his feelings, and accept them as legitimate. Once this has been accomplished, the adolescent will need to acknowledge his complex mixed feelings, and identify ways to reach out for support rather than becoming paralyzed by them. Examples might include self-talk such as, "I'm not the only person who feels this way...It's OK to feel this way...I can get help with this…If I ask for help, they won't reject or hurt me…I can handle this with help."

This step also requires the adolescent to become more familiar with identifying feelings that he has traditionally ignored or minimized, such as helplessness, confusion, powerlessness, frustration, or betrayal. By naming feelings, their power is reduced, and the adolescent is empowered to seek the help needed to begin addressing the feelings, as the following vignette demonstrates:

> Carl came into the therapy session agitated, fidgeting with a pencil, and avoiding eye contact. When he was questioned about his behavior, Carl initially stated that nothing was wrong. As the therapist helped Carl review the first four steps of the cycle, Carl finally stated, "I'm scared to talk to you today." Carl and the therapist talked about his fear until Carl was able to reveal that he had been at a friend's house the night before and watched a pornographic video.

It is important to note that incorporating the pre-offense cycle into the discussion avoids the trap of insisting on the adolescent's cooperation or issuing ultimatums about his participation.

STEP 3 - Try to avoid the feelings
EXIT 3: ADDRESS THE FEELINGS

To break the pattern of avoiding strong feelings, the adolescent must identify and practice a variety of healthy ways to address his feelings. This process includes dealing with the pain involved in beginning to examine strong feelings. If he has learned to cope with difficult feelings through various avoidance techniques, this exit step will be very challenging and painful, and the adolescent and his family will vigorously resist it. Because adolescents perceive they will lose so much safety and security, both individually and within the family system, they often become stuck at this point and need assistance to move beyond this fear.

Coping behaviors at this exit include reaching out to a support person, practicing relaxation techniques, and asking for help. Generally these changes begin in therapy sessions and later generalize to other settings. The intervention here is to normalize the adolescent's feelings, slow the reaction process, and then connect the adolescent with support people. He should start small, first addressing feelings and situations that pose lower risks and limited vulnerability. The following vignette illustrates:

> Once Carl discussed watching the pornography, he reviewed his initial feeling of fear. Carl explored his feelings about talking to the therapist, and examined his fidgeting and avoiding eye contact. The therapist then helped Carl look at other ways he could more directly address his feelings with the therapist, including role playing a number of ways to initiate discussion of a difficult topic.

STEP 4 - Push people away, or attempt to regain power and control
EXIT 4: ASSERTIVELY COMMUNICATE THOUGHTS AND FEELINGS

Many offenders have isolated themselves from others, so it is critical for them to reduce the destructive interpersonal distance that surrounds them. The therapist must assess the adolescent's ability to actively listen, provide accurate feedback, assertively communicate thoughts, ideas, and feelings, and share personal information. The adolescent must explore his many barriers to intimacy, including his feeling of powerlessness, and actively replace them with pro-social skills.Actions at this exit include remaining in communication, finding a safe person with whom to talk, visualizing support people, using self-talk that connects him with others, and preparing to interact appropriately. He must learn assertive communication skills to remain in meaningful relationship with significant others and to participate in a mutually supportive relationship. In treatment, role-playing interactions, practicing new skills, and receiving direct feedback in a safe environment are crucial interventions for accomplishing this task. Daily events and interactions must be utilized in therapy to incorporate these new skills, as demonstrated in the following vignette:

> As Darryl processed the incident of "power-gripping" his therapist's hand in the waiting room, he began to answer questions directly and took responsibility for his actions. He was affirmed for replacing distancing behaviors with clear and direct communication and acknowledging his feelings and concerns in the session. Through this discussion, Darryl recognized that he had been in the offense cycle in the waiting room and was now actively using the relapse prevention exits.

STEP 5 - Choose to dwell on the deviant thoughts and/or sexual feelings
EXIT 5: REPLACE WITH APPROPRIATE THOUGHTS OR ACTIVITIES

When the adolescent has a sexual thought or a desire for sex and power, Step 5 becomes a pivotal point in the offense cycle. Adolescents often identify this as the step at which they either stop themselves or move on in the cycle. The internal process of grooming himself begins here if the adolescent uses abusive sexual fantasies as an imagined resolution to Steps 1 through 4; therefore, the intensity of the exit choices needs to match the intensity of the thoughts.

Many offenders developed sexual fantasies and arousal patterns from pornography, misinformation, or their histories of inappropriate sexual experiences. As this arousal pattern becomes deeply ingrained, it becomes increasingly difficult to change. The National Task Force on Juvenile Sexual Offending (1993) specifies the following assumption: "If arousal patterns indicate significant or fixated interest in deviant and/or other criminal sexual behaviors, it is in the offender's best interest to change or control his arousal" (p. 46). It is important for an adolescent to differentiate between healthy sexual fantasies and deviant ones. If the fantasies and arousal patterns are not replaced, the adolescent remains at risk to reoffend. One residential treatment program emphasizes that appropriate sexual fantasies follow the C.E.R. format; they involve consent, equality, and respect. The offender must take full responsibility for his thoughts as well as his actions. Interventions here include teaching him how to consciously replace the inappropriate sexual fantasy with an appropriate fantasy, visualize a stop sign, consciously use thought replacement, remind himself of the harm to the potential victim and for himself, and talk with a trusted other. The youth needs to identify pleasurable behaviors that are not sexual or abusive which can be substituted for the problematic fantasy. The therapist must help the adolescent engage in new behavior patterns, including exercise and other physical activity, to deal with boredom, free time, or inappropriate thoughts. The following example demonstrates:

> John acknowledged that he frequently masturbated to deviant thoughts and knew that he needed to break this habit. John stated, "I hear people say it's not right for me to do this, but I don't know what else to do." As John discussed his fantasies, the therapist helped him understand the difference between deviant and healthy fantasies. A critical realization that helped John change was that he usually masturbated when he was bored. The therapist helped him identify options for handling boredom, including sports. John later returned to therapy stating that he felt in charge of his fantasies for the first time and joked, "I'm also getting really good at basketball!"

STEP 6 - Convince myself it is OK to offend, begin to plan the offense (groom myself)

EXIT 6: SEE THE PERSON, AND STRENGTHEN THE BARRIERS

The way an adolescent grooms himself through thinking errors and irrational beliefs must be addressed at this exit. The goal is for him to see the child as a human being instead of an object, and develop and strengthen his empathy skills. For offenders with little or no empathy for others, this is one of the most difficult treatment tasks. The adolescent must internalize the child's vulnerability and need for safety in order to successfully intervene in his offense cycle, as illustrated in the following vignette:

> During an assignment on seeing the offense from a child's perspective, Tony was able to view the offense through the eyes of his cousins. Halfway through the assignment, he began to cry and repeated, "What have I done, what have I done?" Once he regained composure, he stated that for the first time, he imagined looking into his cousins' eyes and saw their pain and confusion.

An effective aid in developing empathy is for adolescents to explore their own experiences of trauma. How, when, and whether to incorporate treatment of the offender's own victimization remains open to debate. Certainly, a valid concern is that the adolescent must not use this focus on his own victimization to rationalize or defend his sexual offense behavior. The authors believe it is essential for the adolescent offender to acknowledge and resolve his own victimization as a step in developing empathy for his own experience and for the experience of the child(ren) he molested. Using the pre-offense and offense cycles as the framework for treatment highlights the importance of the adolescent resolving his own victimization. The adolescent's history as a victim and his core beliefs about himself and others influence how he moves through the cycle of offense. A critical part of sexual offender treatment, therefore, is for the offender to experience and resolve the pain of his own victimization. In doing so, adolescents often gain empathy for others. Ryan and Lane (1991) state, "It is also relative to childhood memories that the group members are first able to express some empathy for each other, and through that experience of empathic responses the client becomes able to express some empathy himself for the child he was" (p. 270). The therapist must, however, clarify to adolescents that encountering and resolving feelings about their own trauma experience does not minimize their personal responsibility or justify offending against others.

This is also the point at which the adolescent intervenes in his self-grooming process by replacing his thinking errors with self-talk that connects him with the reality of potential harm to another human being. Thinking of the child by name, thinking of the child's age, and self-talk such as, "I would not want this to happen to my child/brother/sister...Sex is not for a child this young...It would hurt him...This is a person with feelings and needs" are important here. By the later stage of treatment, the adolescent should also be incorporating self-talk that reflects his awareness that being abusive is no longer congruent with his self-image, "I was abusive before, but I cannot be abusive now because I have changed."

The adolescent must be able to verbalize the feelings and reactions of children who have been sexually abused, and to identify the short- and long-term effects on these children. Movies, videos, or books that offer understanding and empathy for children who have been victimized are valuable adjuncts to treatment.

A crucial aspect of an offender's relapse prevention process is the "abstinence violation effect" (AVE), or the thoughts and feelings he experiences when he has a lapse, or an inappropriate sexual urge (Russell, Sturgeon, Miner, and Nelson, 1989). This can be an overwhelming experience for the adolescent and can be a step toward reoffense without intervention. It is crucial that the adolescent be prepared to experience and cope with an inappropriate urge so that he can quickly regain his place in the prevention plan process.

If the adolescent finds himself at the stage of convincing himself it is all right to molest a child, he needs to re-establish and/or increase communication with a trusted other about his advancement through the offense cycle. When he acknowledges to someone that he is in the cycle of offense, he immediately moves toward relapse prevention by breaking through his secrecy and isolation.

***STEP** 7* - Convince myself that I will get away with the sexual offense, break down barriers

***EXIT** 7:* FOCUS ON IMMEDIATE AND LIFELONG EFFECTS FOR SELF AND OTHERS

At this step, the offender must recognize the seriousness of his progression in the cycle and his movement toward sexual perpetration. Because the movement toward offending gains momentum at this stage, the relapse prevention actions must also strengthen. The adolescent must overcome his egocentric focus by calling the potential child victim by name and age, emphasizing the penalties he will face when caught, recognizing that he will not get away with the offense because secrecy cannot be ensured, challenging his distorted notion that this is "the perfect crime," stressing that he is not in total control and needs help, and recognizing that there will be powerful penalties for a repeat offender. Effective relapse prevention at this stage will shift the offender's focus from himself to the immediate and lifelong effects for a child who is sexually abused, as well as for the child's family and the offender's family, as demonstrated in the following example:

For Chris to "remember" the seriousness of his offense and the effect his

> behavior had on others, the therapist helped him change his deviant fantasy by beginning to picture the police entering the room, along with his parents, teachers, friends, and the child's family. As he continued with this train of thought, he was assisted in "playing the tape out" and recalling the negative effects he and the child had experienced after the abuse. Chris broke into a sweat, stating, "It's just not worth it."

Effective relapse prevention at this exit also requires that the offender reduce his isolation. The relapse prevention work done at Step 4 (developing and maintaining intimate relationships, communicating honestly, and talking directly about sexual thoughts and urges) must now be re-emphasized. As the adolescent successfully participates in the therapy group he is able to gain confidence in social interactions that can help him begin to take risks in interacting in new ways with peers outside of group. It can be helpful for the adolescent to carry a list of relapse prevention steps in his wallet, as the following vignette demonstrates:

> Ken talked in group about the previous day when he had experienced a strong urge to peep. He described how he had pulled out his personalized wallet card of relapse prevention exit choices and had used it to remind himself that he hurts people and invades their privacy by peeping. Group members affirmed him for using the exits.

The adolescent must have a firmly established support system and must be willing to actively use it in a meaningful way; at this point in the cycle, it would be extremely difficult to begin developing supports and confidantes.

STEP 8 - Set the stage (select and/or groom the victim)
EXIT 8: STOP! AND REMOVE SELF

At this exit, the adolescent must be able to observe himself, recognize his dangerous behavior, use powerful self-talk to intervene in his cycle, and remove himself from the cycle. This is a crucial last step before sexually offending. Such self-talk as, "I need to remove myself now...I need to get out of here...I need to not be alone...This is a dangerous place for me to be...I am putting this child at risk...If I stop now I won't be arrested" needs to be well-integrated so the adolescent can quickly draw upon these resources now that they are exceedingly necessary. Visual images of juvenile detention or a prison cell, remembering parents'/family's reactions, and recalling the investigating police officer can all help reconnect the adolescent with reality. Specific interventions here include imagining the support and encouragement of the therapist and group members, and calling a crisis or accountability person or a therapist. Use of this exit is demonstrated in the following vignette:

> Greg called his youth care worker from school to say he was experiencing an intense urge for a sexually deviant act and knew that he needed to talk with someone "now."

The adolescent must be sensitive to situations that would place him at high risk to re-offend. This might include being asked to baby-sit or to volunteer with young children, or noticing secluded areas in a park. An effective relapse prevention plan should include developing realistic and workable ways for the adolescent to remove himself from these high-risk situations. Often, role playing these possibilities is helpful. The offender may intellectually know his exits, but he needs to practice how to walk (or talk) through a real-life situation, as demonstrated in the following vignette:

> Todd knew that a high-risk situation would be having a neighbor ask him to baby-sit her children. He knew that if this occurred, he should say no, but he did not want to appear rude or raise too many questions. Therefore, he was asked to role play this possibility. As the role play progressed, Todd received feedback from others in the group regarding what to say. Afterward, Todd stated that he was less anxious and that he could imagine successfully removing himself from this type of situation.

The adolescent needs to take direct actions at this exit, first removing himself from the situation, and then contacting his therapist or a counseling hot line, or confiding in a trusted support person. The offender must decrease his isolation and connect himself with a support person who knows about his offense history so that he has other options to disclosing sensitive information to a stranger at this crisis point. Certainly if no support person is available, the adolescent needs to contact anyone who can help hold him accountable, and he must remove himself from the immediate situation while he determines his next step.

STEP 9 - Sexual offense (pleasure, relief of tension and emotional pain)
EXIT 9: STOP, and LEAVE!

This exit is a concrete reminder to the adolescent that even at this late stage, he is still in charge of not continuing to molest. He still has options. He must remove himself from access to the victim and then reconnect with reality by naming the crisis and acknowledging where he is in his cycle.

It is vital that an adolescent understand that any "justification" for offending is only an excuse. Society does not, nor should it, accept any excuse. Typical attempts to justify an assault include, "I had reached a point of no return and there was nothing I could do about it...I was already in trouble anyway by fondling the child." An offender must accept responsibility for his choices at all times. Intervening at this step requires healthy self-talk, awareness of options, and a willingness to accept the consequences of his behavior up to this point. The adolescent must realize that no matter how difficult it may be to acknowledge that he has reached this step in the cycle, he still can stop the cycle and not continue to reoffend.

A crucial step in the relapse prevention plan at this point is for the adolescent to talk about having reached this step and how he handled his feelings, self-talk, behavior, and choices. It is critical for the adolescent to have a support system whose members (therapist, therapy group, family member, clergy, etc.) will be able to hear the truth, process the re-molestation, and then process how the adolescent made the decisions that led him to this late step of the cycle. This includes examining each step, exploring the progression, discussing each missed exit and how it was bypassed, and re-establishing appropriate exits.

> Lou was left to supervise his 3-year old baby sister "just for a minute" as his mother went to the store. His baby sister went to use the toilet. He followed her in and after she pulled her shorts down he began to fondle her vagina. He had an urge to place his tongue on her genitals. He recalled what happened last time when the police came to the house and he stopped the behavior.

STEP 10 - Self hatred, fear, or guilt (pain returns)
EXIT 10: REGAIN HOPE

When the adolescent has reoffended, he must not handle this step alone. His feelings can become overwhelming, resulting in isolation and despair. It is crucial that he make contact with his support system as soon as possible to acknowledge the crisis. Throughout treatment, clients are encouraged to be honest about urges to re-molest and about their progression in the cycle of offense. When an adolescent discloses that he has reoffended, the therapist must be able to hear him, support the disclosure, and yet hold him accountable for his behavior by reporting the new offense. The adolescent needs to be aware of any report to child protection/law enforcement official or other supervising agency. He must be able to access inner hope that even with having re-molested, intervention at this late stage is still less harmful than continuing in this pattern without disclosure. He also needs to remember how the situation could have become even more out of control had he not stopped his behavior. The following example highlights this:

> Lou exited the bathroom. Thoughts were racing through his head, "I really messed up…She won't tell…Mom will hate me forever…I can't even get over this problem…At least I stopped before I went on."

STEP 11 - Cover-up to self and others (denial and secrecy)
EXIT 11: TALK WITH SAFE PERSON

The relapse prevention options at this step echo the options for the previous step. Again, the adolescent must summon the strength to trust in his support system and reach out, and he must recognize that one incident of re-molestation is either a step toward a pattern of sexually offending or the impetus to becoming seriously committed to relapse prevention. At this point, he needs to understand that the new offending behavior cannot be erased, and what he does next will either prevent his situation from deteriorating further or make things much worse. He will integrate this only if he has learned this lesson with everyday events and small dilemmas. No one can integrate this belief while in a major personal crisis without having first practiced it with smaller, less critical situations. The following vignette demonstrates:

> Lou's self- talk continued, "I can't tell anyone…I'm already in trouble…I know they will put me in detention…Maybe they won't be as hard on me if I tell first…I'll try and tell Mom…She has been listening to me…I promised I would talk to her."

Once an adolescent has developed an individualized relapse prevention plan, he must implement it daily and frequently discuss his conscious use of the exits. It takes constant practice, ongoing support from informed adults, and continued self-vigilance for the adolescent to remain in relapse prevention and not drift back into the distorted thinking and abusive behaviors that characterized his offense cycle. Effective intervention with adolescent sexual offenders requires a systemic approach that involves therapists, collateral staff, parents, and family members, each of whom is knowledgeable about the cycle and relapse prevention exits.

References

National Task Force on Juvenile Offending. (1993). The revised report from the national task force on juvenile sexual offending, of the national adolescent perpetrator network. *Juvenile and Family Court Journal, 44,* 1-120.

Ryan, G.D., & Lane, S. (1991). Integrating theory and method. In G.D. Ryan & S. Lane (Eds.). *Juvenile sexual offending: Causes, consequences, and correction* (pp. 255-298). Lexington, MA: Lexington Books.

Chapter 5

Use of the Cycle in Treatment with Adolescents

> Mark entered treatment and acknowledged that he had continued to sexually offend against several children and had verbally and physically assaulted family members. Mark stated that he had "tried to stay sex-free" but continued to reoffend. During sessions, Mark learned how to place his history, thoughts, feelings, and beliefs into the framework of the cycle of offense. Once his individualized cycle was completed, Mark was able to make sense of his progression into offending and identify exit choices he could make.

Mark discovered what many adolescents experience when they first learn about their individual cycles of offense: that he had choices throughout the cycle, and that specific and practical exits were available. Mark's resolve to remain sex-free had failed because he did not recognize that effective relapse prevention is much more complex than he had envisioned. This chapter discusses the practical application of the Cycle of Offense with Recovery Exits within an overall treatment plan. While this chapter focuses on the use of the offense cycle in treatment, the authors recognize that specialized training and knowledge in sexual abuse treatment and sexual offender treatment is a critical prerequisite in order to integrate this material effectively.

Integrating the Cycle into Treatment

The overall goal of adolescent sexual offender treatment is to hold the adolescent accountable for his abusive behavior and reduce his risk of reoffense. In order to fully integrate relapse prevention into the adolescent's daily life, the cycle must be incorporated into treatment in a comprehensive, consistent, coordinated manner. Each guideline is discussed below:

<u>Comprehensive:</u> When daily events and behaviors are incorporated into the cycle of offense and relapse prevention exits, the result is a more holistic approach to treatment that uses daily events to implement change. It is important for the adolescent to apply his knowledge of his cycle and exits to nonsexual situations and practice new relapse prevention skills extensively. In examining pre-offense behaviors, the adolescent is more open to feedback, as the following vignette illustrates:

> Warren stated he was tired of hearing adults refer to his intimidation of others as "sexual offending behavior." When he learned about his

> cycle of offense, he recognized that his intimidation of others was a part of his cycle. He then was able to examine his abusive behavior less defensively.

Consistent: Once the adolescent begins to integrate the cycle of offense, he needs consistent feedback about his cycle in as many contexts as possible. To effectively treat the adolescent, his therapists must incorporate the cycle into their individual, group, and family modality. Therapists, residential youth treatment specialists, parents, and case managers can provide consistency in the youth's treatment when there is a common philosophical understanding of the cycle and how it is integrated into everyday life. The following vignette demonstrates:

> As Tim's family members learned about his cycle of offense, they were encouraged to incorporate this information into his visits home. During therapy, Tim's grandmother stated that it helped to have a new way to support Tim while he was home, as well as a different way to talk with his therapist and youth treatment specialist about situations that occurred during visits.

The foundational framework of the cycle helps to integrate the separate treatment modalities so that common themes of accountability, self-observation, and non-abusive behavior are emphasized.

Coordinated: As the adolescent begins to outline his cycle of offense in group and individual therapy, on the residential unit, and at home, the adults in his world need to remain in communication with each other about his behavior, using the framework of the cycle and relapse prevention plan. Additionally, his case manager and/or probation caseworker must have an in-depth understanding of the cycle and communicate this to the adolescent during case-review meetings and in written court recommendations, as illustrated in the following example:

> During the case-review meeting, Sam talked about his cycle and how he had used his exits on the unit the previous week. Each staff and family member present at the meeting asked questions about the cycle and affirmed Sam's use of the relapse prevention plan. Later, he told his therapist he was surprised that his caseworker knew what Sam was talking about, and said, "Maybe she really can help me after all."

At times the caseworker may need to educate others in the legal system about the meaning and use of the cycle and exits. To integrate the cycle and relapse prevention plan, maintain consistency, and coordinate with others, each person involved with the adolescent needs to understand the cycle and be able to communicate about it in a meaningful way, as the following vignette demonstrates:

> After a quarterly treatment review meeting, Tom told his therapist that he finally understood why he thought and acted the way he did. He said that since the introduction of the cycle, he finally felt supported, and he could "see some light at the end of the tunnel." His mother stated that learning about the cycle had made her aware of the changes she needed to make in her discipline and communication with Tom.

Introducing the Cycle to Adolescents

The cycle of offense with relapse prevention exits is a complex model and can be visually overwhelming. During the assessment and treatment planning process there are numerous natural opportunities to introduce the language of the cycle without immediately presenting the entire model. Such terms as difficult situation, strong feelings, avoid pain, push people away, convince yourself can very naturally be incorporated into early discussions. Typically, the inclusion of this terminology makes intuitive sense to the adolescent because these are not therapy terms per se; they are common terms that will take on new meaning in treatment. Early in treatment there will be naturally occurring situations where presentation of the cycle is appropriate, as the following vignette illustrates:

> Darryl came into the session stating he didn't have anything to say and that this therapy was a waste of time. The therapist drew an empty pre-offense cycle on a blank sheet of paper and began to write on it while processing what was going on for Darryl (see Table 5.1). Soon the cycle showed what he was saying in **Step 4** ("this therapy is stupid"); what he had experienced that day in **Step 1** (he had to miss a school activity to attend therapy); his strong feelings in **Step 2** (anger at the therapist, his parents, the teachers, his sister, and finally, at himself, embarrassment, frustration, and powerless-ness about attending the event); and the ways he avoided the pain of his feelings in **Step 3** (telling himself he didn't care about that stupid activity anyway and trying to act as if he didn't care).

Table 5.1: Application of Cycle to Daily Events

Cycle Step	*Daily Events*	*Relapse Prevention Behavior*
1: Difficult situation, experience, memory	Miss a school activity to attend therapy	Recognize that the activity was important
2: Strong feelings	Anger at therapist, parents, teachers, sister, himself; embarrassment; frustration; powerlessness	Acknowledge mixed feelings
3: Try to avoid the feelings	Tell himself he doesn't care about that stupid activity anyway; act like he doesn't care	Talk about feelings
4: Push people away, or attempt to regain power and control	Tell therapist, "This therapy is stupid!"	Talk with therapist about the situation

During this session the therapist was able to frame Darryl's experience in a way that helped him get a different perspective on his day, acknowledged his difficult situation, affirmed his feelings and yet held him accountable for his behavior in therapy. Darryl was happy to tell the therapist about the injustice of his experience and about his feelings - the paradox of the cycle is that as soon as he participated in this discussion he was no longer in the cycle and was using relapse prevention exits by engaging in therapy (see Table 5.1). The therapist could then introduce the concept of exits by reinforcing the relapse prevention behaviors Darryl had used during the discussion (acknowledging his feelings, talking about his feelings, and talking with the therapist about the situation). The therapist avoided a power struggle about whether Darryl would participate appropriately in therapy and there was no debate about whether therapy is stupid. Darryl's therapist drew the circle of the offense cycle, but did not identify it and said only, "We'll talk about this part another time." Darryl was curious but aware that there was more to come. Once the concept of the cycle has been introduced in a naturally occurring situation, a comprehensive explanation is appropriate.

Explanation of the Cycle

When introducing the cycle to adolescents, the therapist should help them

Figure 5.1: Framework for Cycle of Offense

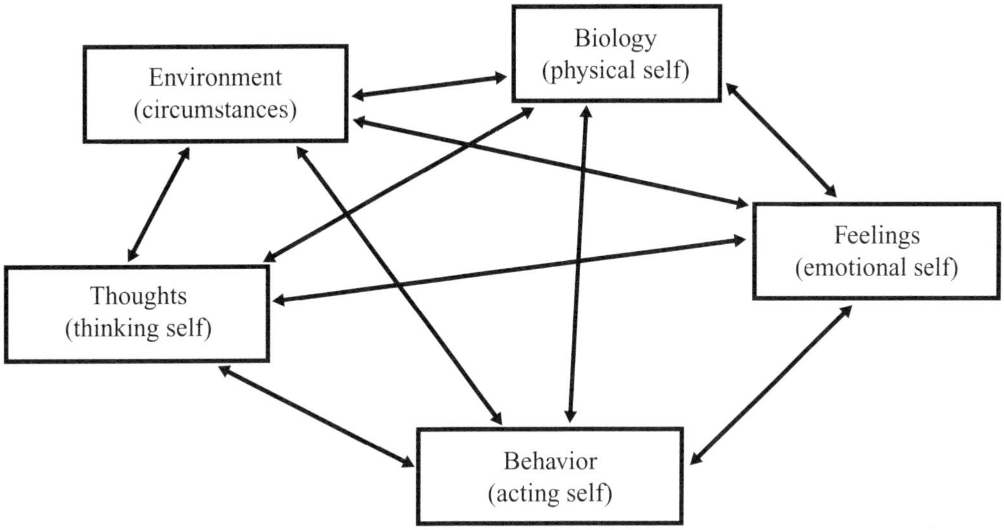

understand the underlying problems or difficulties they have experienced. Problem identification is a key component of intervention in the cycle. Clients who insist they have no problem areas (especially related to their sexual offending) are often difficult, if not impossible, to treat. To engage adolescents in incorporating the cycle, it helps to let them know that the cycle will give them a framework to deal effectively with many of these difficult situations, experiences, or memories.

They need to learn how the cycle can be an effective tool for resolving internal and environmental conflicts. Once they grasp their pre-offense pattern (history, core beliefs, personality development, arousal pattern, etc.), they will have increased understanding of themselves, others, and their environment, and will be able to begin solving their problems more effectively. A cognitive therapy approach to problem solving illustrates how this insight can be gained.

An individualized model helps adolescents understand their difficult situations and use treatment interventions (exits, relapse prevention techniques). The therapist can draw an individualized model that describes a specific problem, and an explicit treatment plan. The following generic dialogue and model are helpful during initial contacts with the client or resident:

> John was having difficulty processing his daily time-outs. He and his therapist discussed John's misbehavior. His behavior was then placed in the framework of the cycle. The therapist introduced the cycle to John using the following diagram:

The therapist stated, "This is a model we use to help understand sexual offenses, stealing, lying, manipulation, etc. All of us live in an environment: family, culture, weather, etc." The therapist then pointed out the environment area on the model. "We are affected by both our current environment, family stress, abuse, lack of supports, and our past environments, whether we have had successes, losses, criticism. In addition, we each have aspects of ourselves such as behaviors, biology, thoughts, and feelings." The therapist pointed to each area on the model.

"I've drawn lines between these aspects because each of these five parts is connected to the others. They all sit inside of our environment and interact with it as well. What we *feel* is closely connected to our *thinking,* our *behavior,* our *physical* health, and our *environment.* For example, you told me that some mornings you feel very down or depressed [writing *depressed* next to *feelings*]. When you are depressed, what is usually going through your mind?" The therapist then wrote these words next to *thinking.* "And when you are feeling and thinking this way, how does your behavior change?" The therapist learned that John showed signs of decreased or withdrawn behavior and wrote these next to *behavior.* "And how do these changes affect your *environment* (family, relationships, etc.)?...So, as you see, changes in one of these areas affect changes in all of the others. And over time, these effects can build as you go round and round.

"Now the good news is that, just as changes in any one of these areas can make you feel worse, changes in any one of these areas can also help you begin to feel better. For example, in the past few weeks, have you had the experience of [pick a positive change most likely for this client]? When that happened, your environment put pressure on you, your behavior changed. Do you remember any changes in your thinking or mood? How about your energy level?...So, as this example shows, if one of these areas changes, the others can change as well. What we will be doing on the unit is, first, learning if this model is true for you; and second, figuring out with you what small changes in your thinking, behavior, environment, physical health, and feelings lead to the biggest improvements in your life. We will also look at the pre-offense cycle and figure out where this information fits."

To help an adolescent understand the pre-offense and offense cycles, the therapist can introduce group and individual therapy exercises. Numerous group exercises are detailed in *A Manual for Structured Group Treatment with Adolescent Sexual Offenders* (Way & Balthazor, 1990).

Helpful Tips/Cautions for Use of the Cycle of Offense

A number of guidelines are useful in effectively integrating the cycle of offense into treatment of adolescent sexual offenders. These include: individualizing the cycle, repetition and integration of cycle concepts, building client ownership of the cycle components, using creativity in incorporating the cycle, providing feedback to the adolescent, and obtaining continuing education. These guidelines are detailed below:

Individualization: This is an important point, but one that often gets lost in treating this population in a group or treatment milieu format. Every offender's history is unique. Some may have sexually abused numerous children; others may have molested one child. Some may have used more aggression or violence in their offense; others discontinued offending at the slightest sign that they would get caught or that the child might tell. Some may have offended within the family system only (incest perpetrators); others may have offended against numerous children in the community. It is important to remember that an elaborate process of gaining insight and awareness must occur for each client in order to prevent relapse, and that even though they have many similar experiences and thought processes, no two offenders are exactly the same. Appendices C and D present typologies of male and female adolescent sexual offenders (Mathews, 1994; O'Brien & Bera, 1986) that detail the primary distinctions for male and female adolescent sexual offenders.

Repetition and integration: Many of the components and theoretical concepts of the cycle are difficult for staff, parents, and therapists to assimilate at first. Most adolescents will have even more difficulty gaining insight into their problems because of limited age, wisdom, experience, intellectual and developmental status, and varying commitment to change. It is therefore vital that exercises, communication, and group discussions be repeated. This helps teens integrate the concepts and framework, and will help them use their exits and relapse prevention skills independently after they leave treatment.

Ownership: Teens must be engaged in the therapeutic process to make long-term gains from any kind of therapy. Adolescent offenders must come to accept that they have a problem that could lead to severe sanctions, including imprisonment, if they do not change and control their behavior. Providing adolescents with respect, a framework for problem solving, and a collaborative working relationship contributes to adolescents' engagement in treatment. Without this shift, they will most likely "jump through hoops" in treatment and will not integrate the nonexploitative thought processes and the ability to identify and intervene in their cycle of offense, both of which are required to help prevent relapse.

Creativity: This is a priority when integrating the cycle into treatment. Adolescents are inundated by computer images and other visual stimuli. Boring lectures and dry presentations will decrease their engagement and fuel resentment and resistance. Make the learning process fun. Remember that although the adolescent committed a serious and harmful crime and has serious lessons to learn, treatment does not always have to be painful to be effective. Balancing confrontation with support is essential.

Feedback: It is helpful for adolescents to hear feedback from all sources in their environment, including therapists, staff, group members, case managers, parents, foster parents, and family members. Give adolescents honest feedback on how they are doing. Model honesty and demonstrate that you can take honest feedback about your behavior as a change agent as well. No one has all the answers. Saying, "I don't know the answer to that question," can be difficult for caregivers. Model a willingness to seek information and engage in problem-solving.

Continuing education: The field of intervention with adolescent sexual offenders is still in its infancy, and new information is emerging constantly. It is important to maintain ongoing contact with other professionals who conduct research on, and treat, adolescent sexual offenders. Membership in professional organizations (e.g.: National Adolescent Perpetrator Network, Association for the Treatment of Sexual Abusers, and American Professional Society on the Abuse of Children); attendance at annual conferences of these organizations; and reading current professional literature (e.g.: Child Abuse and Neglect; Child Maltreatment; Interchange; International Journal of Offender Therapy and Comparative Criminology; Journal of Interpersonal Violence; Sexual Abuse: A Journal of Research and Treatment) enables the clinician to maintain contact with other professionals who work together to prevent further sexual victimization of children.

References

Mathews, R. (1994). Preliminary adolescent female sexual offender typology. In T. Connor, M. Frost, R. Mathews, J. Raymaker, & S. Wolsleger (Eds.), *Adolescent female sexual offenders: A descriptive and comparative study and treatment manual.* Report #SP-93-0053. St. Paul, MN: The St. Paul Foundation..

O'Brien, M., & Bera, W. (1986). Adolescent sexual offenders: A descriptive typology. *Preventing sexual abuse, 1,* 1-4.

Way, I.F. with Balthazor, T.J. (1990). *Manual for structured group treatment with adolescent sexual offenders.* Notre Dame, IN: Jalice Publishers.

Professional Membership Organizations

American Professional Society on the Abuse of Children, 407 S. Dearborn, Suite 1300, Chicago, Illinois, 60605, 312/554-0166.

Association for the Treatment of Sexual Abusers, 10700 S.W. Beaverton-Hillsdale Highway, Suite 26, Beaverton, Oregon, 97005-3035, 503/643-1023.

National Adolescent Perpetrator Network, 1205 Oneida Street, Denver, Colorado, 80220, 303/321-3963.

Chapter 6

Introduction of the Cycle to Collateral Staff and Parents

It is important that treatment of adolescent sexual offenders occurs in a context of clear and direct communication, clear roles and boundaries, and deliberate decision-making so that interactions intentionally promote dynamics that are distinct from dysfunctional family dynamics adolescents may have experienced as they were growing up. Because the therapist has limited contact with the adolescent, it is critical to maintain communication with such caregivers as youth treatment staff, teachers, parents, and foster parents, who have many more hours each day to observe and communicate with the adolescent. These caregivers need to understand that they are an important part of the adolescent sexual offender's treatment process. Because they are critical agents in the adolescent's therapy, their working knowledge of the cycle is crucial in fostering the adolescent's growth. This chapter discusses introduction of the cycle and relapse prevention exits to youth treatment staff and to parents and parent figures (including foster parents and guardians).

Coordinating Use of the Cycle with Collateral Staff

Because adolescent sexual offenders can exhibit fewer sexually acting-out behaviors while in a controlled environment, their daily pre-offense cycle behavior is the primary focus for intervention in their cycle of offense and teaching new relapse prevention behaviors. Youth treatment specialists in residential treatment centers play a key role in providing this feedback and intervention. Residents exhibit pre-offense behaviors many times daily, giving staff ample opportunity to intervene early in the cycle (Steps 1 through 4) and to reinforce relapse prevention behaviors.

The authors recommend specialized training for residential treatment staff. Ryan (1997) details development of "abuse-specific" programming based on the premise that youth in care are at risk for victimization and the milieu must be structured to prevent perpetration of all types. As Ryan (1997) emphasizes, "Abuse is abuse, whether it is physical, sexual, emotional, psychological, or verbal" (p. 407), and is not acceptable. In training youth care staff on use of the cycle in the milieu, it is helpful to relate common problems and behaviors exhibited by residents to the steps of the pre-offense cycle (Steps 1 through 4). This provides a framework to help youth treatment specialists incorporate the cycle into intervention with daily incidents. When introducing the cycle to youth treatment specialists, adequate time is needed for staff to ask questions and practice communicating from a cycle perspective if they are to fully integrate this new framework. Staff need to be reminded that their use of the cycle within the treatment milieu is a significant contribution to the collaborative treatment process. The following vignette illustrates a frequent milieu incident:

> A resident who is normally very active has withdrawn from activities and become argumentative with peers.

The typical staff response might be to use a behavior modification intervention and give the resident a time-out. To integrate the cycle of offense framework, however, the youth treatment specialist instead could help the adolescent connect his behavior to his pre-offense cycle by speaking privately with the resident:

> "I notice you've been quiet all day and just now you were arguing with Ramon. I wonder what's going on for you today?"

Through a dialogue about what is going on for the adolescent, his Step 1 circumstance (difficult situation, experience, or memory) becomes evident for the resident. The youth treatment specialist can help the resident connect Steps 1 through 4 of the offense cycle as they relate to the current situation as detailed in Table 6.1.

Table 6.1: Application of Cycle Steps to Daily Situations

	Cycle Step	*Life Events/Reactions*
Step 1	Difficult situation	Parents no-showed again for their visit
Step 2	Strong feelings	Sad, depressed, disappointed, abandoned
Step 3	Attempts to avoid the feelings	Don't cry, be tough, who cares, doesn't bother me
Step 4	Attempts to push people away	Withdrawing, name calling, sarcasm, bullying

Many other examples of milieu situations can be discussed in the context of the first four steps of the cycle. Staff are encouraged to process incidents regularly until the resident understands how these first four steps apply to the milieu. Once the first four steps have been identified numerous times and are integrated for the resident, the youth treatment staff can use daily opportunities to help the resident recognize his progression through the cycle and replace his unhealthy pattern of avoidance with relapse prevention exit options, as illustrated in the following vignette:

Joe began to realize that much of his misconduct arose from the negative thinking he engaged in when his parents failed to visit as promised. Typically, he would vent his disappointment by bullying his peers. He and his worker then devised a way to intervene at Steps 1 through 3 so that he could avoid the acting out of **Step 4.**

He identified exits at each step. **Step 1** Exits: Talk to my worker, Teri, each time my parents no-show. Write about my parents not visiting, in my journal. **Step 2** Exit: Name my feelings ("I'm really disappointed…I'm really angry at them when they blow me off again!"). **Step 3** Exit: When I'm in therapy, talk about my parents not showing up. **Step 4** Exits: Remind myself not to take this out on the other guys and that it is not their fault. They don't deserve to be treated this way. Bring this problem up in group to see how other guys have handled this problem.

Staff can be reminded that they need to directly challenge the resident's unacceptable behavior while demonstrating empathy for the resident's basic situations and support for his appropriate responses in the early steps of the cycle (Steps 1 through 4). Direct confrontation becomes even more critical when the adolescent's behavior becomes increasingly destructive (Steps 5 through 11). The more residents learn to view the youth treatment specialist as helpful and supportive in the early stages of treatment, the greater the likelihood they will be more honest and less defensive during difficult or intense situations later. As youth care specialists use the framework of the cycle in the milieu, their input at case staffings provides critical insight on the adolescent's treatment progress.

Introducing the Cycle to Parents

When their teen is accused of a sexual offense, parents often feel overwhelmed by "this terrible nightmare." They may also feel angry, shocked, embarrassed, hurt, or responsible, and may even deny parts or all of his behavior. Even if they initially deny their son's offending behaviors, they need to become allies in the treatment process. As Isaac (1986) states, "the majority of treatment providers involved with adolescent sex offenders would agree that family involvement in treatment is seen as pivotal to success." Parents can learn about their teen's cycle of offense and how to support relapse prevention exits in three key ways: participation in a parents' group, discussion in family therapy, and reading specialized literature.

Parents' Group

A parents' group provides support, education, and opportunity for ventilation. Parents have two primary needs that can be met through participation in a parents' group: 1) they need to deal with and resolve their own feelings and reactions, and 2) they need to understand how they fit into their son's treatment. Parents need to be heard and supported empathically if they are to become fully engaged in the therapeutic process. Suggested parent group topics include:

1. Causes and dynamics of sexual offense;
2. Coping with emotional reactions;
3. Empathy for the child who was molested;
4. Relationship of family dynamics to sexual offending;
5. Cycle of offense;
6. High-risk situations and relapse prevention;
7. Preparing for the teen's return home (or determining the nature of a *visiting* relationship).

Steen and Monette (1989) outline detailed topics for a parents' group in their book on community-based treatment for adolescent sexual offenders.

The cycle of offense is best introduced early in the parents' group. This framework provides an intellectual understanding of the dynamics of sexual offense, relates family dynamics to all types of acting out, and offers encouragement for change with the specific relapse prevention exits. Parents quickly relate the steps of the pre-offense cycle to their teen's behavior before and during the time period of the sexual offending and become increasingly engaged in the discussion. The following vignette illustrates:

> Mr. Jones had angrily resisted participating in the parents' group. He maintained that his daughter was just as guilty as his son in the sexual "offense," and he blamed her for not stopping this from happening because she had previously been molested by another older brother, and "she knew this was wrong!" He insisted that his family was different from others and that therapy was not necessary. When the cycle was introduced, he engaged in the discussion, and said that for the first time people were answering his questions, and that he was finally learning something new. Though he continued to resist placing full responsibility for the offense with his son, he was able to identify his son's pre-offense cycle behaviors and attitudes.

It is critical to explain the importance of family history in the teen's personality development. It is helpful to explain that each teen has unique circumstances and history and that it is meaningful to understand how this history contributes to his thoughts, feelings, and behavior patterns. It is important for parents to understand the development of sexuality and the relationship of the cycle to chronic behavior problems (Ryan, 1994). In this way, they can begin to see retrospectively how the child's behavior progressed. Drawing specific attention to the difficult situations the family has experienced, and diagramming those on the cycle assists all family members in understanding the cycle. Parents may become defensive when they hear about "dysfunctional" family dynamics, and it is important to emphasize understanding rather than blaming.

Parents may also be unsure how to be supportive to their son because of their mixed feelings about his offending behavior. The group provides a supportive environment for parents to resolve these feelings and questions. The therapist can present the cycle as a tool to help parents understand their son and remind them that they are experts in identifying their son's behavior, thoughts, and feelings, as well as the environmental circumstances that influence their son's behaviors. As parents resolve questions about their son's cycle of offense and identify his relapse prevention exits, they can become significant allies in the treatment process.

Family Therapy

Family therapy is a critical bridge between the work the adolescent is doing in individual and group sessions, and the work the parents are doing in the parents' group. In family therapy, the therapist can help the adolescent share information about his personalized cycle, as illustrated in the following vignette:

> In the family therapy session, Dan was assisted in explaining to his parents what he had learned about his cycle of offense and exits for his pre-offense cycle. His father, who had sat silently in the session, began to make eye contact with Dan and pointed out that he had noticed Dan being more patient with his younger brother the previous day.

It is important to use the cycle in family sessions and while the adolescent is on home visits. When difficult situations arise at home, these must be processed in family sessions by examining how the situation progressed through the cycle/exits framework. Such a discussion may be facilitated by either the therapist or youth treatment specialist. It is helpful to have numerous copies of the cycle on hand for parents to take home and write on when analyzing difficult situations. These notes must then be discussed during family sessions.

Written Resources

Books that are useful for parents to read and then discuss, either in therapy or in the parents' group, include Pathways: Guide for Parents of Youth Beginning Treatment (Kahn, 1990); Children Who Molest: A Guide for Parents of Young Sex

Offenders (Gil, 1987); and Childhood Sexuality: A Guide for Parents (Ryan & Blum, 1994). In addition, it has been helpful in groups to read first-person accounts from children who have been sexually abused, to help parents understand the feelings and concerns of a child who has been victimized. Parents who struggle with mixed loyalty between their son or daughter who was molested and their teen who has sexually offended against a sibling frequently gain new empathy and insight through this process.

Summary

Collateral staff, parents, and parent figures (foster parents, guardians) are key resources in the adolescent's relapse prevention process. The combined efforts of the adolescent sexual offender, treatment providers, family members, and collateral staff are required to intervene in the cycle of offense and prevent further sexual victimization of children.

References

Gil, E. (1987). *Children who molest: A guide for parents of young sex offenders.* Walnut Creek, CA: Launch Press.

Isaac, C. (1986). Parental involvement in adolescent sex offender treatment. *Interchange,* January, 5-7.

Kahn, T.J. (1990). *Pathways: Guide for parents of youth beginning treatment.* Brandon, VT: Safer Society Press.

Ryan, G. (1997). Creating an "abuse-specific" milieu. In G.D. Ryan, & S. Lane (Eds.). *Juvenile sexual offending: Causes, consequences, and correction* (2nd ed.) (pp. 404-416). Lexington, MA: Lexington Books.

Ryan, G., & Blum, J. (1994). *Childhood sexuality: A guide for parents.* Denver, CO; Kempe Children's Center, University of Colorado Health Sciences Center, Department of Pediatrics.

Steen, C., & Monette, B. (1989). Parent group treatment. In *Treating adolescent sex offenders in the community* (pp. 86-100). Springfield, IL: Charles C. Thomas.

APPENDIX A

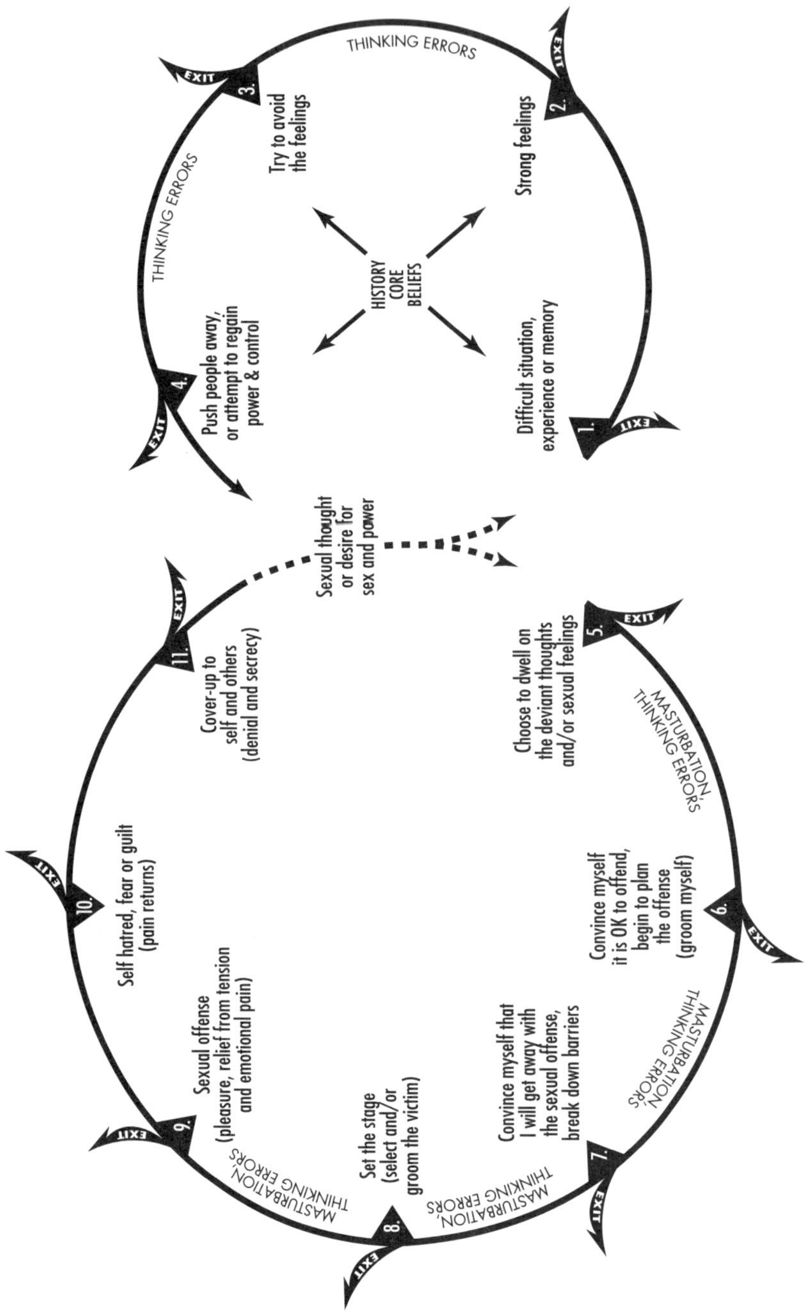

CYCLE OF OFFENSE

APPENDIX B

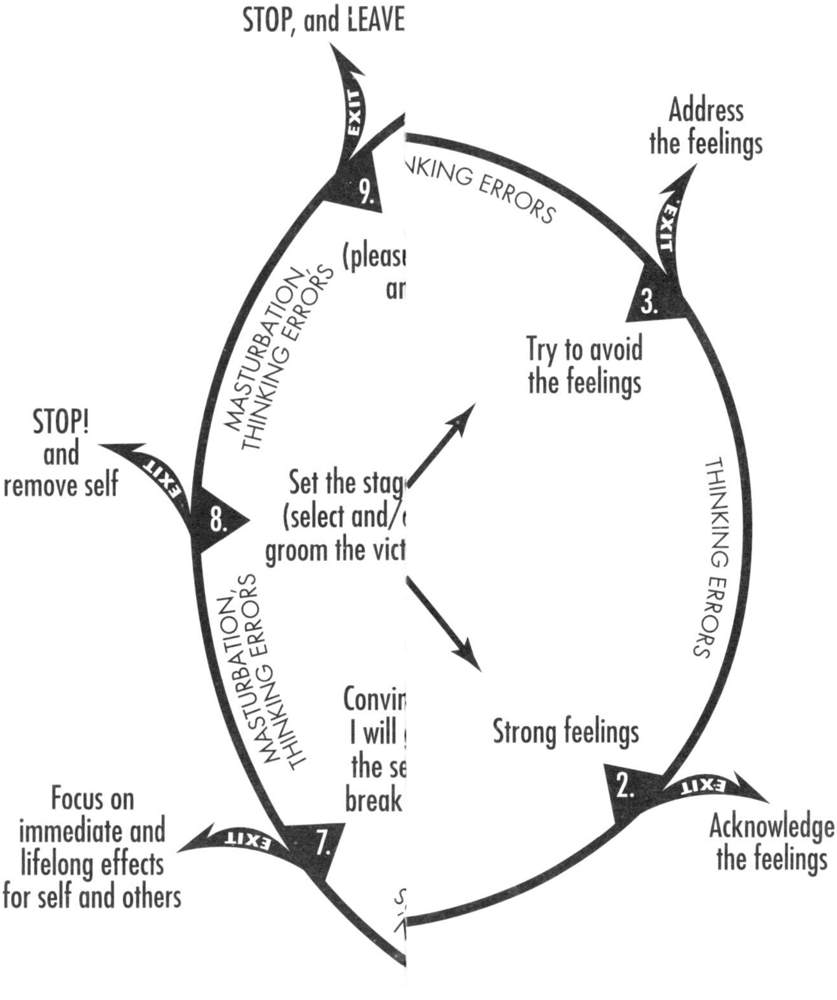

TH RECOVERY EXITS

APPENDIX C:

Typology of Adolescent Sexual Offenders

By Michael J. O'Brien and Walter H. Bera, Program for Healthy Adolescent Sexual Expression (PHASE), Maplewood, Minnesota

Naive Experimenter

1. Tend to be younger adolescents (ages 12 to 15)
2. No previous history of acting-out problems
3. Adequate social skills/socialization
4. Lack of sexual knowledge and experience
5. Sexual events are isolated, opportunistic, exploratory, situational, nonviolent acts with younger children

Under-Socialized Child Exploiter

1. More extensive patterns of sexual behavior with younger children effected through manipulation, enticement, entrapment
2. Chronic social isolation and poor social skills
3. No history of other acting-out behavior
4. Inadequacy, insecurity, low self-worth predominate
5. Family disengaged, father-distant

Pseudo-Socialized

1. Active peers - but manipulative relationships, superficial
2. Narcissistic quality - they play on being special, unique; immunity to other people's pain
3. Sociopathic streak
4. Normal on testing
5. Likes to break rules, not get caught, stealing, etc.
6. Seemingly lots of friends, gifted, successful
7. Magnetic, facile in group, plays at social wellness
8. Lack of intimacy - family has high expectations, little closeness
9. Do well in school, high I.Q., computer programmers, hang around adults

10. Love being viewed as precocious
11. Air of superiority
12. Love to do, dream of very adventurous things
13. Lacking intimacy skills, also their fathers lack intimacy skills while appearing very successful

Sexual Aggressive

1. Use of force or violence in commission of sexual assaults against peers, adults, or older children
2. Socially and sexually active with peer group
3. History of antisocial, acting-out behaviors from early childhood
4. Likely to use alcohol and/or drugs regularly
5. Difficulty handling aggressive impulses
6. Oversensitive to criticism, tense and anxious, emotionally labile
7. Uses primarily denial and projection as defenses
8. Family characterized by chaos, abuse, violence

Sexual Compulsive

1. Engages in repetitive sexually arousing behavior that becomes compulsive, addictive in nature
2. Usually hands-off behaviors such as voyeurism (window peeping), obscene phone calling, exhibitionism, fetish burglary
3. Quiet, socially withdrawn
4. May be studious, tending toward overachievement and perfectionism
5. Constant state of tension and anxiety due to hypersensitivity to failure
6. Inability to express anger appropriately
7. Emotional constraint and anxiety results in tension-reducing acting-out behaviors that involve sexual arousal
8. Behavior becomes patterned, cyclical, and repetitive because it is self-reinforcing
9. Family system rigidly enmeshed with closed external boundaries. Parents may adhere to rigid and fundamentalist religiosity

Disturbed Impulsive

1. Sexual offense is impulsive and signifies acute disturbance or reality testing
2. Offense may be single, unpredictable, uncharacteristic act or pattern of bizarre and/or ritualistic acts
3. Offenses reflect malfunction of normal inhibitory mechanisms due to thought disorder caused by endogenous or drug-induced psychosis

Group-Influenced Offender

1. Sexual offense is an attempt to impress peers, gain approval or acceptance, or prove oneself in peers' presence, e.g., gang rape, "dare" exposing, bathroom abductions
2. Usually no previous history, personality and family characteristics normal

(Reprinted by permission)

APPENDIX D:

Preliminary Adolescent Female Sexual Offender Typology

By Ruth Mathews, Ph.D., L.P., Alpha PHASE, St. Paul, Minnesota

Experimenter/Exploiter

1. Young adolescent
2. Normal background, no history of problem behaviors
3. Offending experimental, outside family, usually in baby-sitting situation, motivated by curiosity, one to few incidents

Coerced/Accompanied/Influenced

1. Females whose offense is initiated by another
2. Their participation is to avoid negative consequences and/or for acceptance

Compulsive

1. Perfectionistic, rigid, and anxious adolescent
2. Family history of rigidity or compulsivity
3. Offending driven by sexual arousal and anxiety reduction
4. Many incidents

Predisposed (by history of abuse)

Adjustment Disordered/Identity Confusion

1. Child or young adolescent - fairly well-adjusted
2. History of some incidents of sexual abuse during childhood, usually outside immediate family
3. Offending occurs either during/following victimization, around onset of puberty or following a trauma (e.g. abandonment, placement)
4. Time-limited childhood offending and/or few adolescent incidents

Lack of Identity Development

1. Child or young identity-disordered adolescent
2. Extensive history of sexual abuse and neglect within the family
3. Offending often occurring between siblings, viewed as somewhat mutual, motivated by a desire for human connection

Learned Deviant Arousal

1. Adolescent with extensive history of sexual abuse, usually by primary caregiver(s), where sexual arousal becomes paired with nurturing/care giving
2. History of indirect strategies to meet needs (e.g., manipulation, undermining, passive aggressive, charming)
3. Offense motivated by paraphilic arousal, unmet childhood affiliation needs and/or bonding, and unresolved arousal to and anger about their own victimization

Disturbed Impulsive

1. Child or adolescent with extensive history of abuse, and unstable and dysfunctional caretaking
2. History of dissociation and/or state-dependent behaviors, severe psychological disorders and problematic behaviors
3. Offending behaviors are linked to own victimization and part of larger profile of psychological disturbance

Sexualized and/or Conduct-Disordered Identity

1. Child or adolescent with an extensive history of abuse
2. History of problematic and/or acting-out behaviors and psychological problems; impairment in empathy for self and others
3. Offending is often extensive, ritualized and linked to own victimization

(Reprinted by permission)

References

Abel, G.G., Mittelman, M.S., & Becker, J.V. (1985). Sex offenders: Results of assessments and recommendations for treatment. In M.H. Ben-Aron, S.J. Hucker, & C.D. Webster (Eds.), *Clinical criminology: Assessment and treatment of criminal behavior* (pp. 207-220). Toronto: M & M Graphics.

Abel, G.G., Osborn, C.A., & Twigg, D.A. (1993). Sexual assault through the life span. In H. Barbaree, W.L. Marshall, & S.M. Hudson (Eds.), *The juvenile sex offender* (pp. 104-117). NY: The Guilford Press.

Abney, V.D., & Gunn, K. (1993). A rationale for cultural competency. *The APSAC Advisor, 6,* 19-22.

Association for the Treatment of Sexual Abusers (1997). *Ethical standards and principles for the management of sexual abusers* (2nd ed.). Beaverton, OR: Author.

Bagley, C., Wood, M., & Young, L. (1994). Victim to abuser: Mental health and behavioral sequels of child sexual abuse in a community survey of young adult males. *Child Abuse and Neglect, 18,* 683-697.

Barbaree, H., Hudson, S.M., & Seto, M.C. (1993). Sexual assault in society: The role of the juvenile offender. In H. Barbaree, W.L. Marshall, & S.M. Hudson (Eds.), *The juvenile sex offender* (pp. 1-24). NY: The Guilford Press.

Becker, J.V. (1990). Treating adolescent sexual offenders. *Professional Psychology: Research & Practice, 21,* 362-365.

Becker, J.V., Cunningham-Rathner, J, & Kaplan, M.S. (1986). Adolescent sexual offenders: Demographics, criminal and sexual histories, and recommendations for reducing future offenses. *Journal of Interpersonal Violence, 1,* 431-445.

Becker, J.V., & Kaplan, M.S. (1988). The assessment of adolescent sexual offenders. In R.J. Prinz (Ed.), *Advances in behavioral assessment of children & families* (pp. 97-118). Greenwich, CT: JAI Press.

Bridges, G.S., Conley, D., Beretta, G.R., Engen, R.L., Price-Spratlin, T., Rankin, M., & Steen, S. (1993). *Racial disproportionality in the juvenile justice system: Final report.* Olympia, WA: Washington State Commission on African American Affairs and Management Services Division/Department of Social Services.

Clark, M. (1995, March). *Uniting adolescent sex offenders and their families through treatment.* Keynote Address presented at the National Adolescent Perpetrator Network Meeting, St. Louis, MO.

Fehrenbach, P.A., Smith, W., Monastersky, C., & Deisher, R.W. (1986). Adolescent sexual offenders: Offender and offense characteristics. *American Journal of Orthopsychiatry, 56,* 225-233.

Finkelhor, D., Araji, S., Baron, L., Browne, A., Peters, S.D., & Wyatt, G.E. (1986). *A sourcebook on child sexual abuse.* Newbury Park, CA: Sage Publications.

Ford, M.E., & Linney, J.A. (1995). Comparative analysis of juvenile sexual offenders, violent nonsexual offenders, and status offenders. *Journal of Interpersonal Violence, 10,* 56-70.

Gil, E. (1987). *Children who molest: A guide for parents of young sex offenders.* Walnut Creek, CA: Launch Press.

Gilby, R., Wolf, L., & Goldberg, B. (1989). Mentally retarded adolescent sex offenders: A survey and pilot study. *Canadian Journal of Psychiatry, 34,* 542-548.

Gilgun, J.F., & Connor, T.M. (1990). Isolation and the adult male perpetrator of child sexual abuse: Clinical concerns. In A.L. Horton, B.L. Johnson, L.M. Roundy, & D. Williams (Eds.), *The incest perpetrator: A family member no one wants to treat* (pp. 74-87). Newbury Park, CA: Sage Publications.

Gomes-Schwartz, B., Horowitz, J.M., & Calderelli, A.P. (1990). *Child sexual abuse: The initial effects.* Newbury Park, CA: Sage Publications.

Griffiths, D.M., Quinsey, V.L., & Hingsburger, D. (1989). *Changing inappropriate sexual behavior: A community-based approach for persons with developmental disabilities.* Baltimore: P.H. Brookes Publishing Co.

Huizinga, D., & Elliott, D.S. (1987). Juvenile offenders: Prevalence, offender incidence, and arrest rates by race. *Crime and Delinquency, 33,* 206-223.

Hunter, J.A., Lexier, L.J., Goodwin, D.W., Browne, P.A., & Dennis, C. (1993). Psychosexual, attitudinal, and developmental characteristics of juvenile female sexual perpetrators in a residential treatment setting. Journal of Child and Family Studies, 2, 317-326.

Isaac, C. (1986). Parental involvement in adolescent sex offender treatment. *Interchange,* January, 5-7.

Kahn, T.J. (1990). *Pathways: Guide for parents of youth beginning treatment.* Brandon, VT: Safer Society Press.

Kahn, T.J., & Chambers, H.J. (1991). Assessing reoffense risk with juvenile sexual offenders. *Child Welfare, 70,* 333-345.

Kahn, T.J., & Lafond, M.A. (1988). Treatment of the adolescent sexual offender. *Child and Adolescent Social Work, 5,* 135-148.

Knopp, F.H. (1984). *Remedial Intervention in Adolescent sex offenses: Nine program descriptions.* Brandon, VT: Safer Society Press.

Knopp, F.H., Freeman-Longo, R., & Stevenson, W.F. (1992). *Nationwide survey of juvenile and adult sexual offender treatment programs and models.* Brandon, VT: Safer Society Press.

Knopp, F.H., & Lackey, L.D. (1987). *Female sexual abusers: A summary of data from 44 treatment providers.* Brandon, VT: Safer Society Press.

Krisberg, B., Schwartz, I., Fishman, G., Eisikovits, Z., Guttman, E., & Joe, K. (1987). The incarceration of minority youth. *Crime and Delinquency, 33,* 173-205.

Lab, S.P., Shields, G., & Schondel, C. (1993). Research note: An evaluation of juvenile sexual offender treatment. *Crime and Delinquency. 39,* 543-553.

Lakey, J.F. (1995). Thinking errors in adolescent sex offenders. *Treatment Today,* p.31.

Lane, S. (1994). The cycle. *Interchange,* June, 1-18.

Lane, S. (1991). Sexual abuse cycle. In G.D. Ryan, & S. Lane (Eds.), *Juvenile sexual offending: Causes, consequences, and correction* (pp. 103-142). Lexington, MA: Lexington Books.

McGarrell, E.F. (1993). Trends in racial disproportionality in juvenile court processing: 1985-1989. *Crime and Delinquency, 39,* 29-48.

Marshall, W.L., Laws, D.R., & Barbaree, H.E. (1990). *Handbook of sexual assault: Issues, theories, and treatment of the offender.* New York: Plenum Press.

Mathews, R. (1994). Preliminary adolescent female sexual offender typology. In T. Connor, M. Frost, R. Mathews, J. Raymaker, & S. Wolsleger (Eds.), *Adolescent female sexual offenders: A descriptive and comparative study and treatment manual.* Report #SP-93-0053. St. Paul, MN: The St. Paul Foundation..

Mathews, R., Hunter, J.A., & Vuz, J. (1997). Juvenile female sexual offenders: Clinical characteristics and treatment issues. *Sexual Abuse: A Journal of Research and Treatment, 9,* 187-199.

Murphy, W.D., Coleman, E.M., & Haynes, M.R. (1983). Treatment and evaluation issues with the mentally retarded sex offender. In J.G. Greet & I.R. Stuart (Eds.), *The sexual aggressor: Current perspectives on treatment* (pp. 22-41). New York: Van Nostrand Reinhold Co.

National Adolescent Perpetrator Network. (1993). The revised report from the national task force on juvenile sexual offending, of the national adolescent perpetrator network. *Juvenile and Family Court Journal, 44,* 1-120.

O'Brien, M.J. (1989). *Characteristics of male adolescent sibling incest offenders: Preliminary findings.* Brandon, VT: Safer Society Press.

O'Brien, M., & Bera, W. (1986). Adolescent sexual offenders: A descriptive typology. *Preventing Sexual Abuse, 1,* 1-4.

Regoli, R.M., & Hewitt, J.D. (1991). *Delinquents in society: A child-centered approach.* New York: McGraw-Hill, Inc.

Rogers, C.M., & Tremaine, T. (1984). Clinical intervention with boy victims of sexual abuse. In S. Greer & I.R. Stuart (Eds.), *Victims of sexual aggression: Men, women, and children* (pp. 91-104). New York: Van Nostrand Reinhold.

Russell, K., Sturgeon, V.H., Miner, M.H., & Nelson, C. (1989). Determinants of the abstinence violation effect in sexual fantasies. In D.R. Laws (Ed.), *Relapse prevention with sex offenders* (pp. 63-72). New York: The Guilford Press.

Ryan, G. (1997). Creating an "abuse-specific" milieu. In G.D. Ryan, & S. Lane (Eds.). *Juvenile sexual offending: Causes, consequences, and correction* (2nd ed.)(pp. 404-416). Lexington, MA: Lexington Books.

Ryan, G.D. (1989). Victim to victimizer: Rethinking victim treatment. *Journal of Interpersonal Violence, 4,* 325-341.

Ryan, G., & Blum, J. (1994). *Childhood sexuality: A guide for parents.* Denver, CO; Kempe Children's Center, University of Colorado Health Sciences Center, Department of Pediatrics.

Ryan, G.D., & Lane, S. (1991). Integrating theory and method. In G.D. Ryan, & S. Lane (Eds.), *Juvenile sexual offending: Causes, consequences, and correction* (pp. 255-298). Lexington, MA: Lexington Books.

Ryan, G.D., & Lane, S. (1991). *Juvenile sexual offending: Causes, consequences, and correction.* Lexington, MA: Lexington Books.

Ryan, G.D., & Miyoshi, T. (1990). Summary of a pilot follow-up study of adolescent sexual perpetrators after treatment. *Interchange,* January, 6-8.

Saunders, E.B., & Awad, G.A. (1988). Assessment, management, and treatment planning for male adolescent sexual offenders. *American Journal of Orthopsychiatry, 58,* 571-579.

Schwartz, I.M. (1989). *(In)justice for juveniles: Rethinking the best interests of the children.* Lexington, MA: Lexington Books.

Sermabeikian, P., & Martinez, D. (1994). Treatment of adolescent sexual offenders: Theory-based practice. *Child Abuse and Neglect, 18,* 969-975.

Showers, J., Farber, E.D., Joseph, J.A., Oshins, L., & Johnson, C.F. (1983). The sexual victimization of boys: A three-year survey. *Health Values: Achieving High-Level Wellness, 7,* 15-18.

Smith, W.R. (1988). Delinquency and abuse among juvenile sexual offenders. *Journal of Interpersonal Violence, 3,* 400-413.

Smith, H., & Israel, E. (1987). Sibling incest: A study of the dynamics of 25 cases. *Child Abuse and Neglect, 11,* 101-108.

Steen, C., & Monette, B. (1989). Parent group treatment. In *Treating adolescent sex offenders in the community* (pp. 86-100). Springfield, IL: Charles C. Thomas.

(1991). *Uniform crime reports for the United States.* Washington, D.C.: U.S. Department of Justice.

(1993). *Uniform crime reports for the United States.* Washington, D.C.: U.S. Department of Justice.

Ward, K.M., Heffern, S.J., Wilcox, D.A., McElwee, D., Dowrick, P., Brown, T.D., Jones, M.J., & Johnson, C.L. (1992). *Managing inappropriate sexual behaviors: Supporting individuals with developmental disabilities in the community.* Anchorage, AS: Alaska Specialized Education and Training Services, Inc. (ASETS).

Wasserman, J., & Kappel, S. (1985). *Adolescent sex offenders in Vermont.* Burlington, VT: Vermont Department of Health.

Way, I.F. with Balthazor, T.J. (1990). *Manual for structured group treatment with adolescent sexual offenders.* Notre Dame, IN: Jalice Publishers.

When kids molest kids. *Newsweek, (1992, March 30),* 68-70.

Worling, J.R. (1995). Adolescent sibling-incest offenders: Differences in family and individual functioning when compared to adolescent nonsibling sex offenders. *Child Abuse and Neglect, 19,* 633-643.